LIVER DISEASE AND LABORATORY MEDICINE

LABORATORY MEDICINE SERIES

Series Editors: Gwyn McCreanor BSc, MSc, PhD, MRCPath
William Marshall MA, PhD, FRCP, FRCPath

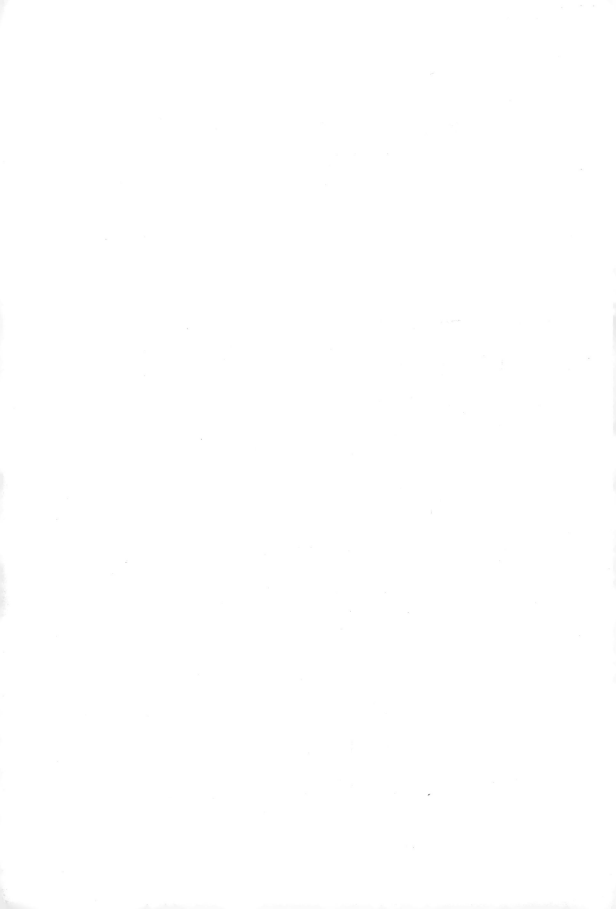

Liver Disease and Laboratory Medicine

Ian McFarlane, BSc, PhD, DSc (Med), FRCPath
Consultant Clinical Scientist and Honorary Senior Lecturer, Institute of
Liver Studies, King's College Hospital, London, UK

Adrian Bomford, MB BS, MD, FRCP
Reader in Hepatology and Honorary Consultant Physician, Institute of
Liver Studies, King's College Hospital, London, UK

Roy Sherwood, BSc, MSc, DPhil
Consultant Clinical Scientist and Honorary Senior Lecturer, Clinical
Biochemistry, King's College Hospital, London, UK

ACB VENTURE PUBLICATIONS

with generous support from Abbott Diagnostics Division

ACB VENTURE PUBLICATIONS
Chairman - David Burnett

LABORATORY MEDICINE
Series Editors - Gwyn McCreanor and William Marshall

British Library Cataloguing in Publication Data

A catalogue record for the book is available from the British Library

ISBN 0 902429 10 8 ACB Venture Publications

Printed by KSC Printers Ltd, Tunbridge Wells, Kent

Preface

Liver disease impacts virtually all areas of the clinical laboratory. The differential diagnosis of liver disease has expanded significantly over the past 20 years as our understanding of autoimmune liver disease has increased and the viral hepatitis alphabet has grown. Developments in diagnostic techniques, particularly in imaging, has greatly improved diagnostic accuracy. Several of the more sophisticated techniques that have been developed (e.g. ultrasonography, angiography, endoscopy and percutaneous liver biopsy) require highly trained personnel for their adminstration and interpretation and/or are invasive procedures that cannot be frequently repeated. Furthermore, the availability of many of these techniques is largely confined to specialist centres and, for initial diagnosis and subsequent follow-up of patients with liver disease, the majority of clinicians still have to rely on laboratory tests performed by local laboratory services. The developments in treatment of patients with liver disease, particularly the growth in liver transplantation, have produced a group of patients for whom long-term monitoring is required, often at local hospitals rather than the transplant centres.

During many years of lecturing to medical and paramedical undergraduate and postgraduate students, we have been faced with a continuing problem in recommending suitable simple texts on laboratory testing in liver disease. The information is available in several excellent comprehensive texts on clinical hepatology, but can be difficult to locate. There seemed to be a need for a relatively small volume in which the essentials of the laboratory investigation of hepatic disorders could be drawn together for easy reference. Ten years ago a book on the Laboratory Investigation of Liver Disease was produced by Drs Johnson and McFarlane from King's College Hospital. The growth in knowledge in the field of liver disease over the past ten years has led to the need to substantially update the information contained in that book. This book is not designed to be a technical manual. Rather, it is intended as an interpretative guide to the laboratory diagnosis and monitoring of liver disease. We have deliberately excluded the field of liver histology as this is adequately covered in suitable specialist texts.

We are grateful to our colleagues at King's College Hospital and to our editors, Gwyn McCreanor and William Marshall, for their advice and criticism of early drafts of this text. Finally, we are grateful to Alan Sherwood for preparation of many of the diagrams used in the book.

Ian McFarlane
Adrian Bomford
Roy Sherwood

ACKNOWLEDGEMENTS

The authors are grateful to the following for permission to reproduce or adapt material for certain figures used in the text::

O'Grady JG, Schalm SW, Williams R. Acute liver failure: Redefining the syndrome. Lancet 1993; 342: 273-5 (Figure 1.7)

Tredger JM, Sherwood RA. The Liver: New functional, prognostic and diagnostic tests. Ann Clin Biochem 1997; 34: 121-41 (Figure 5.6)

Bernuau J, Goudeau A, Poynard T et al Multivariate analysis of prognostic factors in fulminant hepatitis B. Hepatology 1986; 6: 648-51 (Figure 9.1)

O'Grady JG, ALexander GJM, Hayllar KM, Williams R. Early indicators of prognosis in fulminant hepatic failure. Gastroenterology 1989; 97: 439-45 (Figure 9.1)

Contents

Chapter 1

Introduction to Liver Disease

THE LIVER

The liver is the largest solid organ in the body. In adults, it weighs 1.0-1.5 kg and its size is maintained in relatively constant proportion to body weight, increasing or decreasing as weight is gained or lost. It is comprised of a large right lobe and a smaller left lobe, which nestle against the diaphragm under the rib cage in the upper right quadrant of the abdomen (Figure 1.1), and it is the only organ that has the capability to regenerate completely (to exactly the right size) after it has been damaged or following a partial hepatectomy.

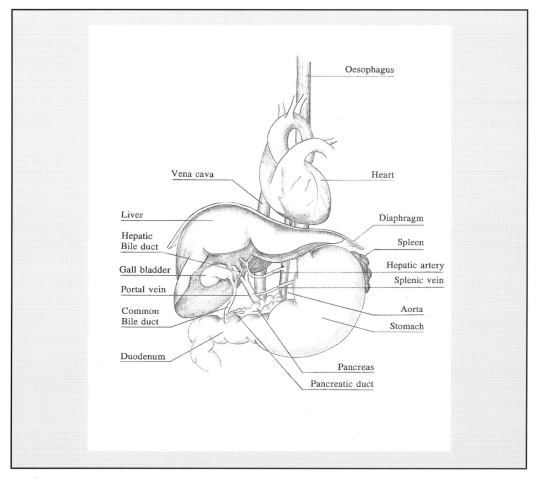

Figure 1.1 Anatomy of the liver.

It is arguably the most important organ in the body, performing numerous complex functions:

- through the processes of glycogenesis, glycogenolysis, gluconeogenesis and ketogenesis it maintains the body's energy supply,
- it manufactures many of the plasma proteins, including most of the blood clotting factors,
- it contributes to digestion through the production of bile,
- it is the major site of lipid metabolism,
- through ureagenesis it has a significant role in hydrogen ion homeostasis,
- it plays a key role in the detoxification of ammonia and of xenobiotics, such as drugs, ethanol and other toxic substances, by transforming them into relatively harmless compounds that can be excreted in the urine or bile.

Parenchymal cells (hepatocytes) comprise some 80% of the cells in the liver and perform the main metabolic functions. However, other important (but less well understood) functions are performed by the non-parenchymal cells: endothelial lining cells, Ito cells (fat-storing), and the Kupffer cells (modified macrophages) and pit cells (related to natural killer cells) which are thought to play a role in defence against infection.

STRUCTURE
The liver is an extremely vascular organ and is unique in having a dual blood supply, receiving blood via both the hepatic artery and the portal vein. The total volume of blood passing through the liver each day is in excess of 2000 litres, about 80% of which is delivered via the portal vein. The latter is fed by a network of vessels carrying blood mainly from the intestines (the splanchnic circulation) and from the spleen (via the splenic vein). The remaining 20% is delivered via the hepatic artery, which branches directly from the aorta and carries 80% of the oxygen delivered to the liver. The hepatic artery and portal vein enter the liver on its underside (Figure 1.1) and then branch repeatedly to form a network of arterioles and venules that run in channels, the portal tracts, and deliver the blood directly to the hepatocytes.

Hepatocytes are arranged in single-cell thick sheets or 'plates' (Figure 1.2), supported by a fine meshwork of a collagenous material known as reticulin, overlying which are fenestrated endothelial lining cells. Hepatocytes are bathed by the blood flowing through the sinusoids on each side of the plates - a construction that allows for rapid exchange of substances between the blood and the cells. Blood then exits the liver via branches (terminal hepatic venules) of the hepatic veins, which empty into the vena cava.

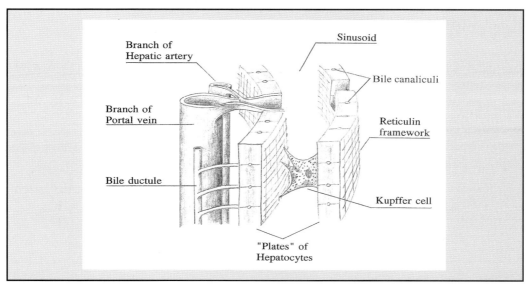

Figure 1.2 Illustration of the internal architecture of the liver showing 'plates' of hepatocytes

The liver has an acinar (glandular) structure that can be visualised either as groups of portal tracts surrounding a terminal hepatic venule (also called a central vein) or groups of central veins surrounding a portal tract (Figure 1.3).

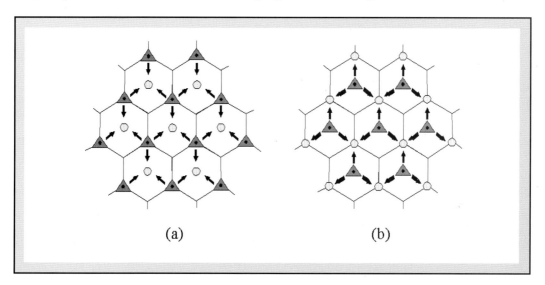

Figure 1.3 Diagrammatic representation of the acinar structure of the liver. The acini may be visualised either: (a) as groups of portal tracts (triangles) surrounding central veins (circles), or (b) as groups of central veins surrounding portal tracts. In either event, normal blood flow is unidirectional across the lobules, from portal tracts to central veins.

Acini, more commonly termed liver lobules, represent microcirculatory units that perform essentially similar functions throughout the liver. Within each lobule, two main zones can be defined: a periportal (afferent or proximal) area which is perfused with blood rich in oxygen and metabolic substrates, and a perivenular (efferent or distal) area around the central vein which is perfused with blood that has been altered during its passage through the lobule and is relatively depleted in oxygen and many metabolites but is enriched in CO_2 and other excretory products. Between these two zones is an ill-defined area (the intralobular area) which is intermediate in terms of the composition of the perfusing blood.

Metabolic zonation of the liver

Periportal zone	Perivenular zone

OXIDATIVE ENERGY METABOLISM
   Fatty acid oxidation
   Citric acid cycle
   Respiratory chain
	XENOBIOTIC METABOLISM

GLUCONEOGENESIS	GLYCOLYSIS
CHOLESTEROL SYNTHESIS	LIPOGENESIS
AMINO ACID UTILIZATION	KETOGENESIS
BILE FORMATION	
AMMONIA DETOXIFICATION	
UREA SYNTHESIS	GLUTAMINE SYNTHESIS

Figure 1.4 **Metabolic zonation in the liver**

FUNCTIONAL HETEROGENEITY

Awareness of this feature is important in understanding mechanisms of liver damage because, although all hepatocytes contain the same genomic information, they do not all perform the same functions. Due to the sequential exchange of solutes between hepatocytes and the blood as it flows from portal tracts to central veins, marked changes in oxygen tension and concentrations of solutes occur across the lobules. As a consequence, oxidative functions of the liver tend to be performed by hepatocytes in the periportal area (where the oxygen tension in the afferent blood is high), while cells around the central vein are generally more involved in metabolic processes that can operate at lower oxygen tensions (Figure 1.4). Similarly, ammonia entering the lobule at high concentration in the afferent blood is rapidly detoxified by conversion to urea mainly in the periportal area but there is a scavenging mechanism, involving conversion to glutamine by glutamine synthase in a few hepatocytes around the central vein, to remove final traces of ammonia before the blood leaves the liver. This functional microheterogeneity is regulated partly by changes in concentrations of solutes and the differential action of hormones through induction of enzymes and up or down regulation of expression of cell surface receptors involved in the various metabolic pathways. However, it is likely that other factors are involved because there is evidence that some hepatocytes constitutively express certain enzymes, and/or preferentially express certain cell surface receptors, in a manner that is not directly influenced by their microenvironment, and that the microinnervation of the lobule may play an important (but as yet poorly understood) role.

The clinical significance of this microheterogeneity can be illustrated in the context of xenobiotic metabolism. Many, potentially toxic, foreign substances such as drugs are detoxified by oxidation, reduction or hydrolysis, often followed by conjugation with glucuronic acid, sulphate or glutathione. Perivenular hepatocytes have a greater capacity for these transformations due to their higher activities of the main drug-metabolising enzymes, the cytochrome P-450 monooxygenases, and subsequent conjugation with glucuronic acid also appears to be greater in this zone. However, sulphate conjugation involves the action of sulphotransferase, which is located to a greater extent in the periportal area. The family of glutathione transferase enzymes catalyse detoxification reactions between reduced glutathione and electrophilic compounds or hydrogen peroxide. Although activities of the glutathione-S-transferases are higher in the perivenular area, the concentration of their substrate, glutathione, is highest in the periportal area where glutathione conjugation is favoured. Furthermore, the action of the cytochrome P-450 monooxygenases often leads to the production of highly reactive species including hydrogen peroxide, superoxides and hydroxyl radicals that can initiate chain reactions leading to extensive lipid and organic peroxide formation and consequent cell damage. These toxic species are inactivated via superoxide dismutase, catalase and glutathione peroxidase. The latter (like its substrate, glutathione) is present at highest level in the periportal area, which benefits from its protection. This pattern probably explains why many xenobiotics induce fatty changes and cell damage predominantly in the perivenular area.

BILE FORMATION

Bile is a complex mixture of cholesterol, cholesteryl esters, proteins, bile salts (mainly taurocholate and glycocholate) and bile pigments - mainly bilirubin (the breakdown product of haemoglobin from effete red blood cells). Disruption of the delicate balance between these components can lead to their precipitation and the formation of gallstones. Before conjugation bilirubin is practically insoluble in aqueous solution and in the blood, it is normally tightly bound to albumin. On entering the hepatocyte, this complex dissociates and the bilirubin is rendered soluble by conjugation with glucuronic acid by UDP-glucuronosyltransferase.

Although all hepatocytes can produce bile, it is predominantly formed in periportal cells. Bile is actively secreted via the bile canaliculi. These are microvillous indentations of the contiguous portions of the plasma membranes between adjacent hepatocytes that form channels which lead into collecting ductules. Bile then flows through ducts of increasing size that run in the portal tracts and carry the bile out of the liver in a countercurrent direction to the afferent blood flow. Bile leaves the liver via the hepatic bile ducts and is stored in the gallbladder. The action of food entering the duodenum triggers secretion of the hormone cholecystokinin, which stimulates the gallbladder to contract and express bile into the common bile duct and thus into the duodenum through the sphincter of Oddi. Release of secretin and pancreozymin is also activated by food in the duodenum. These two hormones stimulate the flow of pancreatic juice. The latter is secreted via the pancreatic duct, which joins the common bile duct just before the sphincter, and mixes with the bile as it enters the duodenum. Pancreatic juice and bile play an essential role in digestion. Bicarbonate in the pancreatic juice neutralises gastric acid, providing an optimal pH for the action of pancreatic enzymes (lipases, endopeptidases and amylase), while the detergent action of bile salts is essential for emulsification of fats to aid their digestion by the pancreatic lipases. Bile salts are reabsorbed in the intestine and returned via the systemic circulation to the liver. This enterohepatic circulation of bile salts has important clinical implications (see below).

DISEASES OF THE LIVER

Diseases of the liver are classified according to aetiology (Figure 1.5). For clinical purposes, a sub-classification defining the stage of the disease process (acute, subacute, chronic, etc.) and the pathological state of the liver (assessed clinically, histologically or radiologically) is usually included. For example, rather than simply stating that a patient has alcoholic liver disease, a diagnosis of acute alcoholic hepatitis or alcoholic cirrhosis imparts more precise information for

Aetiology of liver disease		
Viral	*Biliary tract obstruction*	*Parasitic*
Hepatitis viruses A to E	Gallstones	Schistosomes
Epstein-Barr virus	Strictures	Liver flukes
Cytomegalovirus	Sclerosing cholangitis	Toxocara sp.
Arboviruses	Biliary atresia	Tapeworms
Arenaviruses	Tumours	Leptospira sp.
Metabolic	*Vascular*	*Protozoal*
Haemochromatosis	Budd-Chiari syndrome	Amoebiasis
Wilson disease	Portal vein thrombosis	Kala-azar
Hereditary hyperbilirubinaemias	Veno-occulusive disease	Malaria
Autoimmune	*Toxic/drug-induced*	*Bacterial*
Autoimmune hepatitis	Alcohol	Tuberculosis
Primary biliary cirrhosis	Drugs	Pyogenic liver abcesses
Neoplastic	*Miscellaneous*	*Cryptogenic*
Primary	Polycystic liver disease	(cause unknown)
Secondary	Congenital hepatic fibrosis	

Figure 1.5 Example of the classification of liver disease according to aetiology

clinical management and for assessing prognosis. On the other hand, the liver has only a limited number of responses to various pathological insults, and the signs, symptoms and management problems in patients with hepatic disease often relate more to the liver pathology than to the aetiology of the condition. Thus, patients with cirrhosis suffer much the same range of problems regardless of the aetiology of the cirrhosis. Once the aetiology, stage and state of the disease has been established, therefore, management often revolves around dealing with the clinico-pathological problems independently of aetiology.

CHOLESTASIS AND JAUNDICE
Cholestasis is the term used to describe the consequences of failure to produce and/or excrete bile. The failure may be related to problems in secretion of bile by hepatocytes ('intrahepatic cholestasis') due to parenchymal damage of any cause or in the flow of bile out of the liver ('extrahepatic cholestasis') due to obstruction. In either event the net result is the accumulation of (mainly conjugated) bilirubin in the blood, leading to jaundice. As the jaundice develops, it is usually accompanied by darkening of the urine (due to urinary excretion of water soluble bilirubin and its metabolites) and, because of the lack of bile excretion into the duodenum and therefore of bile pigments (which are responsible for the characteristic colour of faeces), stools become lighter in colour and tend to float (due to their high

content of undigested fat). Jaundice may also be due to excessive haemolysis, as occurs in the many different forms of haemolytic anaemia, in which case the excess bilirubin in the blood is predominantly unconjugated and does not appear in the urine.

Thus, three types of jaundice are usually recognised: hepatocellular (intrahepatic cholestasis), obstructive (extrahepatic cholestasis) and haemolytic. Strictly speaking, extrahepatic (obstructive) cholestasis is not necessarily a disease of the liver because the obstruction may occur anywhere between the hepatic ducts and the sphincter of Oddi. However, prolonged extrahepatic obstruction can often lead to intrahepatic damage and so-called 'biliary-type' cirrhosis (see below).

ACUTE HEPATITIS AND ITS SEQUELAE

Acute inflammation of the liver, associated with hepatocyte damage, is most often caused by viruses or toxins (including drugs and alcohol), although there are many other causes and the mechanisms of cell damage vary. Symptoms depend on the severity of the process and the individual's response to the damaging agent.

There are three main possible outcomes (Figure 1.6):
- complete resolution,
- progression to chronic liver disease of varying severity,
- acute liver failure (ALF).

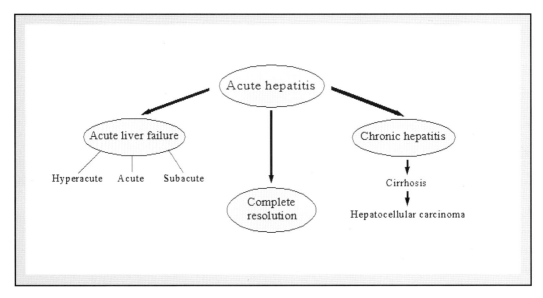

Figure 1.6 The potential outcomes of acute hepatitis

The latter implies the development of severe hepatic dysfunction within 6 months of the first symptoms and in the absence of any pre-existing liver disease. The characteristic clinical feature is the development of encephalopathy (see below), usually in association with severe coagulopathy (due to the failure of damaged hepatocytes to synthesise clotting factors). When these features develop very quickly (within 8 weeks of the onset of symptoms), ALF used to be described as fulminant hepatic failure - a rare but often fatal condition. However, because onset of symptoms is often ill-defined, recent recommendations are that ALF should be classified as hyperacute, acute or subacute, according to the time from the first appearance of jaundice to the first signs of developing encephalopathy (Figure 1.7).

Classification of acute liver failure			
	Hyperacute	**Acute**	**Subacute**
Time of onset of jaundice to first signs of encephalopathy	0 - 7 days	7 - 28 days	5 - 26 weeks
Aetiology			
Paracetamol	100%	-	-
Other drugs	35%	53%	12%
Hepatitis A	55%	31%	14%
Hepatitis B	63%	29%	8%
Hepatitis C	14%	39%	48%
Features			
Cerebral oedema	+++	++	+
Coagulopathy	+++	+++	+
Bilrubin elevation	+	+++	+++
Prognosis	Moderate	Poor	Poor

Adapted from O'Grady et al, Lancet 1993; 342: 273-5

Figure 1.7 Classification of acute liver failure

HEPATIC ENCEPHALOPATHY

Hepatic encephalopathy is a condition that can be associated with either acute or chronic liver failure. Developing encephalopathy begins with symptoms of a mild confusional state (Grade 1) and may progress through various stages of increasing disorientation and reduced consciousness (Grades 2 and 3) to coma (Grade 4). Early symptoms include a characteristic inability to hold the outstretched hands in dorsiflexion ('hepatic flap') and a typical peculiar odour on the breath ('hepatic fetor'). It is reversible with improvement in liver function but its progression is usually a poor prognostic sign. The pathogenesis is not well understood. Undoubtedly, the inability of the failing liver to remove the many potentially neurotoxic substances (including ammonia) from the blood is a factor but it is likely that increased sensitivity of the brain (due to changes in the blood-brain barrier) and additional toxic substances arising from necrotic liver tissue also contribute.

CHRONIC LIVER DISEASE
The distinction between acute and chronic liver disease is a temporal one. The usual yardstick is persistence of signs (clinical or biochemical) and/or symptoms for more than 6 months, but the initial onset of the disease is often difficult to define. For example, primary biliary cirrhosis (Chapter 6) and haemochromatosis (Chapter 4) have no recognisable acute phases and develop slowly and with few, if any, symptoms over many months or years, while in chronic hepatitis C (Chapter 3) the initial viral infection is often clinically silent and the disease may not become apparent for 20 or 30 years.

Chronic hepatitis was previously classified on histological criteria as chronic active hepatitis (CAH), a severe form with a high propensity to progress to cirrhosis and/or liver failure, and chronic persistent hepatitis (CPH) - a more benign form that was considered to progress only occasionally to CAH. The latter was characterised histologically by a dense inflammatory infiltrate spilling out of the portal tracts into the periportal areas, with disruption of the limiting plates (interfaces) that surround the portal tracts, and piecemeal necrosis of periportal hepatocytes. In severe cases, the necroinflammation extended further into the lobules ('lobular hepatitis'). CPH was defined as mild inflammation confined to portal tracts, with no disruption of the interfaces or hepatocellular necrosis. These terms became adopted as clinical entities associated with a poor or good prognosis, respectively. However, in recent years it has become recognised that they merely represent the extremes of what is probably a continuous spectrum of morphological changes in the liver and that one can frequently convert to the other, either spontaneously or in response to treatment, and that cirrhosis can develop without apparently passing through a CAH stage. This has led to the recommendation that use of these terms be discontinued. Today, the classification is based on aetiology together with more precise descriptions of the histological features and assessment of severity, and 'CAH' has been supplanted by the term 'interface hepatitis'.

CIRRHOSIS

As noted above, the liver has a remarkable capacity to regenerate after it has been damaged. Following a single, short-lived, insult it can often recover completely with virtually normal architecture. When the cause of the damage persists, however, as for example in chronic viral infection, the capacity of the regenerative process to keep pace with the liver cell death may be exceeded. A number of events ensue. Firstly, the reticulin framework that supports the liver cell plates collapses and may condense to form fibrous scar tissue. At the same time, resident stellate cells (Ito cells, perisinusoidal cells, lipocytes) which promote fibrogenesis become activated, partly through the influence of various cytokines. As the fibrous tissue deposition becomes more extensive, bridges of scar tissue form between adjacent portal tracts and/or between portal tracts and central veins (Figure 1.8).

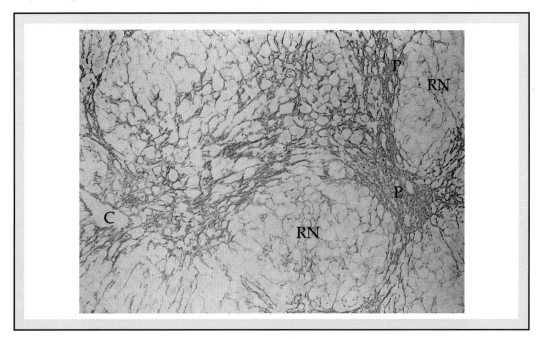

Figure 1.8 Section of a liver biopsy from a patient with cirrhosis stained with silver to reveal the reticulin frame work within the liver nodule: P=portal tract; C=central vein; RN=regenerative nodule. Note that the normal architecture is severely disrupted to the extent that a central vein cannot be identified.

Foci of regenerating liver cells form 'regenerative nodules' within the fibrotic areas. These events lead to disruption of the acinar architecture and, consequently, of the normal passage of blood across the liver lobules which, in turn, creates areas of relative deficiency in oxygen and nutrients, and can result in further cell death. This is the irreversible end result of any chronic process which involves recurrent waves of cell death and attempts by the liver to regenerate. The rapidity with which it develops depends in large part on the severity and duration of the necroinflammation and varies widely with different aetiologies of liver disease. A 'pre-cirrhotic' stage in which there is extensive fibrosis but no definite nodule formation is often recognised and may persist for many years before progressing to an established cirrhotic pattern.

Cirrhosis is also the end result of diseases such as primary biliary cirrhosis and primary sclerosing cholangitis (Chapter 6), in which there is progressive destruction of the intrahepatic bile ducts, and it can also develop when there is prolonged (usually partial) extrahepatic biliary obstruction. The mechanisms underlying this 'biliary type' cirrhosis are poorly understood but it is likely to be at least partly due to damage to hepatocytes which are unable to effectively secrete bile and to episodes of interface hepatitis at various stages.

Even when frank cirrhosis has developed, there may be sufficient surviving parenchyma for the liver to continue to perform most of its normal functions, and patients may have no untoward symptoms. In such cases, their cirrhosis is said to be 'well compensated'. In other instances, there may be rapid deterioration ('decompensation') with the development of complications and liver failure. The severity of cirrhosis is usually described by the use of Pugh's modification of Child's classification (Figure 1.9). Patients with long-standing cirrhosis are at increased risk of developing hepatocellular carcinoma (see below).

Child Pugh classification			
	Grade		
	1	**2**	**3**
Ascites	Absent	Slight	Moderate
Encephalopathy	None	1 and 2	3 and 4
Albumin (g/L)	> 35	28 - 35	< 28
Bilirubin (μmol/L)	< 25	25 - 50	> 50
Prothrombin time (seconds prolonged)	1 - 4	4 - 6	> 6

Figure 1.9 Pugh's modification of Child's classification for assessing severity of liver disease

PORTAL HYPERTENSION

Portal hypertension is the term used to describe increased blood pressure in the portal vein. This may be due to increased resistance to the flow of blood through the liver as a result of the extensive fibrous tissue deposition in the liver in patients with cirrhosis but there is evidence that other factors, independent of hepatic resistance, play a role. The consequence of this increased portal pressure is that blood is diverted into the lower-pressure systemic circulation, particularly the veins around the upper part of the stomach and the lower end of the oesophagus, but also in the rectum and the anterior abdominal wall (portal-systemic shunting). The gastric and oesophageal vessels, which are relatively thin walled, become varicose. Additionally, the spleen often becomes enlarged (hypersplenism) due to the back pressure created in the splenic vein, which drains into the portal vein.

The clinical importance of portal hypertension is three-fold:

- there may be catastrophic haemorrhage from the oesophageal or gastric varices,
- the natural filtering and detoxifying functions of the liver are bypassed and this increases the risk of development of hepatic encephalopathy,
- hypersplenism is associated with sequestration of white blood cells in the spleen and the resulting neutropenia and thrombocytopaenia in the systemic circulation decreases the patient's resistance to infections.

In recent years, the development of endoscopic techniques for injecting sclerosants to obliterate, or for ligation to choke off, the varices, and pharmacotherapy with β-blockers to reduce portal pressure, has led to significant reductions in the mortality due to variceal haemorrhage.

ASCITES

Ascites is the excessive accumulation of extracellular fluid in the peritoneal cavity. Most frequently, it is a complication of advanced cirrhosis but ascites can also develop during acute liver failure in the absence of cirrhosis as well as in a number of non-hepatic conditions (Figure 1.10).

The precise mechanisms are still not fully understood, but the primary event in cirrhosis is probably sodium retention (due in part to secondary hyperaldosteronism), compounded by hypoalbuminaemia and fluid is localised to the peritoneal cavity because of portal hypertension. Thus, the urine may become virtually sodium free and, as long as sodium intake exceeds output, fluid will continue to accumulate. The tendency to retain salt is present before ascites actually develops and a sudden increase in dietary salt intake may lead to ascites, which may spontaneously clear when the salt intake is restricted. Ascites does little harm in itself and the main aim of therapy (bed rest, salt restriction, diuretics, paracentesis) is to make the patient more comfortable. However, careful monitoring is required because of the risk of serious complications if there is developing renal failure. Otherwise, the main potential complication is spontaneous bacterial infection of the ascites. This usually leads to fever, rigors, and colicky abdominal pain, together with hepatic decompensation, but in up to a third of cases the peritonitis may be silent and the only indication is progressive deterioration of hepatic function. The major differential diagnosis is 'non-spontaneous' bacterial peritonitis due to bowel perforation.

Figure 1.10 Causes of ascites

Causes of ascites	
Primary hepatic disease	**Non-hepatic diseases**
Cirrhosis	Abdominal malignancy
Budd-Chiari syndrome	Cardiac failure
Portal vein thrombosis	Constrictive peritonitis
Acute liver failure	Peritonitis (especially tuberculous)
	Malnutrition
	Pancreatic disease

RENAL FAILURE

Renal failure is an ever-present risk in patients with advanced cirrhosis but can also occur in severe acute liver disease and is likely to precipitate encephalopathy. Onset is usually indicated by rising plasma concentrations of creatinine and urea and usually, but not invariably, decreased urine output. Hyperkalaemia is a particularly lethal complication. A major clinical problem is an idiopathic form of renal failure known as the 'hepatorenal syndrome' which is usually associated with advanced disease, ascites and encephalopathy. This is distinct from renal failure in other situations where renal and liver disease co-exist: polycystic disease, infections such as leptospirosis, circulatory failure, and the immune complex glomerulonephritis associated with viral hepatitis. Renal failure may also develop when cirrhotic patients become fluid depleted, and following surgery to relieve obstructive jaundice. The latter syndrome is caused by acute tubular necrosis, but the mechanism is unknown.

The characteristic feature of hepatorenal syndrome, also known as 'functional renal failure' is that the kidneys are histologically normal, i.e., there is disturbance of function but not of structure, and the usual appearances of acute tubular necrosis are not seen. The precise pathogenesis is unknown, but the immediate precipitating event is an intense renal vasoconstriction leading to decreased renal blood flow and reduced glomerular filtration rate. In addition to reduced urine output and rising plasma creatinine and urea concentrations the characteristic feature, which distinguishes it from acute tubular necrosis, is the dramatic increase in sodium retention.

NEOPLASTIC DISEASES OF THE LIVER

Primary neoplasms of the liver may arise from malignant transformation of any of the normal hepatic cells (Figure 1.11). Benign tumours are very rare. Metastatic (secondary) deposits of tumours arising in other organs (especially the intestinal tract, lungs and breast) are, however, much more common that primary hepatic malignancy. Hepatocellular carcinoma (often confusingly termed hepatoma) is by far the most common hepatic malignancy. Hepatocellular carcinoma (HCC) usually arises against a background of cirrhosis and is thought to be a consequence of de-differentiation and transformation of cells in regenerating nodules.

Tumours of the liver			
		Tumour	
	Cell	Benign	Malignant
Hepatocyte		Hepatic adenoma	Hepatocellular carcinoma Hepatoblastoma
Bile duct		Cholangioma	Cholangiocarcinoma
Endothelial		Haemangioma	Angiosarcoma

Figure 1.11 Benign and malignant tumours of the liver according to cell of origin.

On average it takes about 20 years for a tumour to appear after cirrhosis has first developed. Overall, patients with long-standing cirrhosis of any cause have a 10-20% risk of developing HCC. However, the risk is higher in men than in women and the incidence varies widely with aetiology. HCC is very rare in patients with cirrhosis due to autoimmune hepatitis and develops most commonly in cirrhosis due to hereditary haemochromatosis or chronic hepatitis B or C viral infection. There is evidence that these viruses (especially hepatitis B) may have oncogenic potential. Environmental agents such as the potent carcinogen aflatoxin (produced by a mould that grows on improperly stored groundnuts) are also important factors in the development of HCC. Alcohol (which is not itself carcinogenic) also seems to increase the risk. Patients with cirrhosis who consume alcohol regularly develop HCC more frequently and over a shorter time period than those who abstain.

Most primary tumours of the liver are difficult to diagnose at an early stage because the liver has such a huge capacity to function normally. Their development often becomes apparent only when they have grown large enough to cause mechanical problems through invading or otherwise obstructing major blood vessels or bile ducts, or to cause pain - by which time the tumour may already have metastasized to other organs and there is little that can be done. Tumours in other organs around the liver (particularly the pancreas) may also cause problems directly by mechanical obstruction of the extrahepatic bile ducts. Hepatoblastomas are rare (usually slow growing) tumours of childhood but, again, may not be diagnosed until they reach a significant size in early adulthood. Tumours of the bile ducts are also quite rare except in patients with primary sclerosing cholangitis, who have a relatively high risk of developing cholangiocarcinoma.

Chapter 2

Biochemistry and haematology tests

INTRODUCTION

The liver has many diverse functions and it is, therefore, unlikely that any single biological marker would be able to detect all abnormalities of liver disease. Many candidate markers have been put forward as tests of liver disease, but standard practice is for the initial assessment of liver disease to incorporate a profile of biochemical and haematological 'liver function tests (LFTs)'. The aim of such tests is to answer three questions. In a particular patient, is liver disease present, and, if so, what is the nature and severity of the disease? Negative results of LFTs are also valuable as they indicate a low probability of significant disease.

The first question is pertinent in situations where the clinical evidence of liver disease is lacking, for example, during the early phase of viral hepatitis or during therapy with a potentially hepatotoxic drug. The second is clearly important before treatment can be started, or a prognosis given. For optimal therapy an accurate diagnosis is desirable and the increase in the number of diagnostic techniques (immunological, virological and imaging) has improved the diagnostic efficiency in liver disease. It is important to recognise that the standard LFTs offer limited quantitative information and measure dysfunction or damage rather than function. Nevertheless, the vast experience that has accrued with these tests, their simplicity and low cost have meant that the standard LFTs constitute a significant proportion of the workload of a typical laboratory. LFTs have a valuable role in monitoring the progress of established liver disease and in assessing the response to treatment. It is important, however, to be aware of the limitations of their use to avoid over interpretation and potential mismanagement.

The standard LFTs are usually considered to include the following groups:

- bilirubin measurements in blood and urine,
- plasma enzyme activities: commonly used are the aminotransferases, alkaline phosphatase and γ-glutamyl transferase,
- plasma proteins: total protein, albumin and, by subtraction, globulins,
- measures of clotting: prothrombin time.

This chapter covers the physiological basis of the biochemical and haematological tests used in the initial assessment of liver disease, their use in clinical practice and the patterns of abnormality within the panel of LFTs as seen in specific conditions.

BILIRUBIN AND BILE PIGMENT METABOLISM

METABOLISM OF BILIRUBIN

Bilirubin is a yellow-orange coloured pigment derived from haem (Fe-protoporphyrin IX). Metabolic studies using radio-labelled precursors of bilirubin show that there are two peaks of production. The first, between 0 and 2 days after isotope administration, represents breakdown of haem containing proteins such as catalase, myoglobin and the cytochromes, and accounts for 20% of bilirubin production. A second peak at 120 days is attributable to the destruction of effete red blood cells; this represents the major source of haem and ultimately bilirubin. The initial and rate limiting step in the production of bilirubin is the oxidation of haem to biliverdin; this is followed by reduction to bilirubin, with the production of an equimolar amount of carbon monoxide and ferric iron. About 500 µmol (275 mg) of bilirubin is produced each day. The production of bilirubin takes place in the reticuloendothelial system, predominantly in the liver, spleen and bone marrow. The bilirubin produced binds tightly, but reversibly, to albumin (Ka = 10^{-9}) in a molar ratio of 1:1 at normal concentrations, but additional binding sites with lower affinity are recruited in hyperbilirubinaemic states. Unconjugated bilirubin is insoluble in water at physiological hydrogen ion concentrations because of intramolecular hydrogen bonds which prevent ionization of the two terminal carboxylic acid groupings. Binding to albumin prevents extrahepatic (particularly brain) uptake of the lipid soluble, potentially toxic, unconjugated bilirubin and enables transport to the liver. Albumin is capable of binding up to 400 µmol/L of bilirubin but other compounds such as thyroxine and some drugs can compete for the binding sites, potentially displacing bilirubin.

In the liver the albumin-bilirubin complex dissociates and bilirubin enters the hepatocyte across the sinusoidal membrane by a carrier-mediated process where it binds to cytosolic proteins, mainly ligandin (glutathione S-transferase B). Bilirubin is conjugated in the endoplasmic reticulum with glucuronic acid by the enzyme uridine diphosphogluconate glucuronosyl transferase to form mono- and di-glucuronides that are water soluble. The bilirubin conjugates are excreted in the bile, probably via an energy-dependent, carrier-mediated process to overcome a significant concentration gradient. Some conjugates will be deconjugated by glucuronidases of bacterial origin and, being lipid soluble, will be reabsorbed into the hepatic portal system establishing an enterohepatic circulation (Figure 2.1). Bile pigments reaching the colon undergo bacterial degradation to urobilinogen and stercobilinogen. An extrahepatic circulation also exists for these compounds, a small fraction reaching the systemic circulation and being excreted in urine. The remainder is excreted in the faeces. Some urobilinogens oxidize spontaneously to stercobilin, an orange-brown pigment responsible for stool colour.

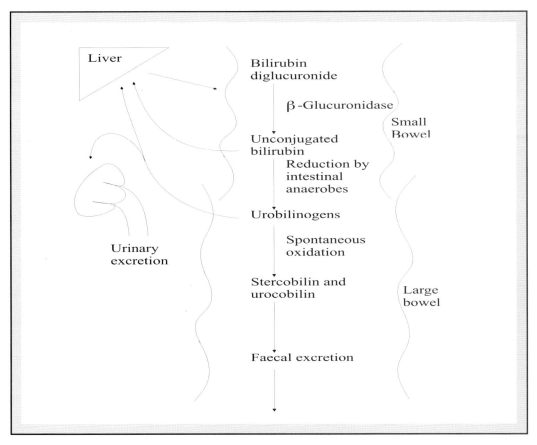

Figure 2.1 The enterohepatic circulation of bilirubin

MEASUREMENT OF BILIRUBIN AND ITS FRACTIONS

Conjugated bilirubin reacts with diazotized sulphanilic acid to produce an azobilirubin, a coloured compound which can be easily quantified. Due to the intramolecular hydrogen bonding in unconjugated bilirubin the reaction with sulphanilic acid cannot occur unless the bonds are disrupted by the addition of alcohol or caffeine. The conjugated bilirubin fraction has, therefore, been termed 'direct reacting' and the unconjugated fraction 'indirect reacting'. By carrying out the reaction with and without the addition of alcohol or caffeine it is possible to measure total and conjugated bilirubin respectively. An estimate of the unconjugated fraction is obtained by subtraction of the conjugated bilirubin result from the total bilirubin. Measurement of bilirubin fractions is important in clinical practice, particularly in assessing neonatal jaundice, but the limitation of the analytical methodology must be recognised. At total plasma bilirubin concentrations less than 50 μmol/L the test is not totally reliable because of underestimation of conjugated bilirubin, whilst at high total bilirubin concentrations the conjugated fraction is overestimated. Urinary bilirubin can be reliably detected by 'dipstick' testing and its presence indicates hepatic or biliary tract dysfunction. Urinary urobilinogen can also be measured, but in this case it is decreased concentrations which indicate failure of biliary excretion and hence biliary tract obstruction. Accurate measurement of low concentrations of urobilinogen is difficult and the test has been superseded by imaging techniques.

HYPERBILIRUBINAEMIA

In more than 95% of the apparently normal adult population, the plasma bilirubin concentration is below 20 μmol/L and this can be considered the upper limit of the reference range. Above 50 μmol/L, hyperbilirubinaemia can often be detected as jaundice by experienced observers, and when in excess of 100 μmol/L may be apparent to patients themselves or their relatives. The amount of bilirubin in the plasma of an individual is determined by the balance between production and clearance. Although less than 500 μmol/L of bilirubin is produced each day, the normal liver is capable of conjugating up to 2 mmol/day. This large functional reserve is one reason why plasma bilirubin is a relatively insensitive test for liver disease, remaining normal until substantial hepatocyte loss or dysfunction has occurred. The absolute concentration of plasma bilirubin is of little help in establishing a diagnosis but can be valuable in monitoring disease progression and in assessing response to treatment. Whilst quantitation of the conjugated and unconjugated fractions is important in the assessment of neonatal jaundice in the adult patient it is seldom necessary unless intra-vascular haemolysis is suspected.

HAEMOLYTIC JAUNDICE

The production rate of bilirubin is directly related to the red cell survival time and, as this becomes shorter in haemolytic disorders, so the plasma bilirubin concentration rises in direct proportion. The maximum compensatory increases in red cell production that the bone marrow can achieve is about eight-fold and this corresponds to a plasma bilirubin concentration of not more than 75 μmol/L. Thus the common chronic haemolytic disorders present with mild unconjugated hyperbilirubinaemia with no bilirubin in the urine. Plasma aminotransferase activity (of red cell rather than liver origin) may be slightly elevated and an increased reticulocyte count is characteristic.

There are two situations in which plasma bilirubin concentrations above 75 μmol/L may occur in haemolytic anaemia. First, when there is associated liver damage and clearance is compromised, as can occur in acute alcoholic hepatitis. Second, in acute haemolytic crisis (in sickle cell anaemia, for example), the production rate of bilirubin can exceed the maximum rate of hepatic clearance. In these situations an increasing proportion of the plasma bilirubin will be conjugated and the haemoglobin concentration will fall as red cells are destroyed faster than the bone marrow can replace them.

NEONATAL JAUNDICE

Normal full-term babies may be jaundiced from the second to the eighth day of life, and premature babies for longer. This 'physiological' jaundice, in which the plasma bilirubin concentration seldom exceeds 100 µmol/L, is unconjugated and is attributable to a combination of factors: increased production and impaired uptake or conjugation of bilirubin together with increased reabsorption from the gut. Jaundice detectable on the first day of life or persisting longer than 7-14 days is pathological, as is conjugated hyperbilirubinaemia at any time.

If the unconjugated bilirubin concentration exceeds 300 µmol/L in full-term infants, there is a significant risk of kernicterus (brain damage due to uptake of unconjugated bilirubin) and treatment by phototherapy or exchange transfusion is indicated. Kernicterus occurs when the maximum binding capacity of plasma albumin for bilirubin is exceeded. In pre-term low birthweight babies, kernicterus may occur at lower bilirubin concentrations, both because of low albumin binding capacity and immaturity of the blood-brain barrier. Although various anions bind to albumin and could theoretically displace bilirubin, only maternal salicylate or sulphonamide use has been demonstrated to increase the risk of kernicterus by releasing bilirubin.

In pathological neonatal jaundice it is essential to ascertain whether the jaundice is due to unconjugated or conjugated bilirubin as the differential diagnosis for each type is considerably different (Figure 2.2). Many of the causes of neonatal jaundice, including the hereditary conjugated hyperbilirubinaemias, are covered in later chapters of this book. One condition, not discussed elsewhere, in which early diagnosis greatly improves the prognosis is extra hepatic biliary atresia (EHBA)

EHBA is characterised by an inability to excrete bile due to obstruction, destruction or absence of the extra hepatic bile ducts and affects one in 14,000 live-born infants in the UK. EHBA must be considered in any infant with jaundice persisting or developing after 14 days of age. The plasma bilirubin at presentation is typically in the range 100-200 µmol/L with more than 60% in the conjugated form. Plasma aminotransferases and GGT are elevated, usually 2 to 10 times normal. Plasma alkaline phosphatase is usually elevated but plasma albumin is normal in the early stages. As EHBA is a cause of conjugated jaundice, bilirubin is present in the urine, whilst the stools have little or no pigmentation. Unless treated, the biliary obstruction results in the progressive development of cirrhosis which can eventually decompensate. If identified early, a hepatic portoenterostomy (Kasai procedure) can be carried out with a successful resolution of jaundice in 70-90% of infants operated on before 8 weeks of age. Further delay in making the diagnosis often results in sufficient progression of the cirrhosis to make surgery impossible and liver transplantation becomes the only option. The definitive diagnosis is made by liver biopsy and technetium-labelled hepatobiliary imaging e.g. HIDA (2, 6-dimethylphenylcarbomylmethyliminodiacetic acid) scan. Two other conditions that present with a similar picture to EHBA and also benefit from surgical intervention are choledocal cysts and spontaneous bile duct perforation.

Causes of neonatal jaundice	
Unconjugated	Haemolytic disorders e.g. blood group incompatibility red cell enzyme deficiency Increased red cell mass e.g. placental or twin-twin transfusion Hypoxia Galactosaemia Fructosaemia Meconium retention Hereditary unconjugated hyperbilirubinaemias
Conjugated	Infections - bacterial or viral Biliary atresia Cryptogenic Genetic conditions - hereditary conjugated hyperbilirubinaemias Endocrine - hypothyroidism Chromosomal Vascular abnormalities Total parenteral nutrition

Figure 2.2 Causes of neonatal jaundice

THE AMINOTRANSFERASES

PHYSIOLOGY AND BIOCHEMISTRY

These enzymes, previously designated as 'transaminases', catalyse the transfer of an amino group from an α-amino acid to an α-oxo acid. The two most widely measured for clinical purposes are aspartate aminotransferase (AST) and alanine aminotransferase (ALT). Although commonly used as tests of hepatocellular damage, these enzymes have a wide tissue distribution. As well as the liver, AST is found in the heart, skeletal muscle, kidney, brain, erythrocytes and lung. ALT has a similar distribution but activities are much lower in tissues other than the liver. The relative contributions of the particular tissues to normal plasma concentrations of aminotransferases are unknown, but the total activity must reflect the net effect of production and clearance. When a pathological increase occurs, it will clearly be dependent not only on the nature of the cellular injury but also on the plasma half-life of AST and ALT which are about 48 and 18 hours respectively. ALT is a cytosolic enzyme, whereas AST exists in both a cytosolic and a mitochondrial form (mAST). mAST is synthesized under control of nuclear DNA in the cytoplasm as 'pre-mAST' and rapidly transferred across the mitochondrial membranes during which it is converted to mature mAST.

USE IN CLINICAL PRACTICE
The increased activities of the aminotransferases in plasma from patients with liver disease are presumed to originate from necrotic or damaged hepatocytes. The aminotransferases are sensitive tests of hepatocyte damage and may be elevated in asymptomatic individuals with viral hepatitis. Generally speaking their specificity for liver disease increases with the degree of elevation of the enzyme activity. Above 10 times the upper limit of the reference range, providing rhabdomyolysis or muscular dystrophy can be excluded, primary hepatocyte damage is indicated so that the hepatic pathology will be some form of acute or chronic hepatitis. Values below this are non-specific and need to be considered alongside other test results. For instance, release of AST from skeletal muscle or from the heart, rather than the liver, can be clearly identified by measurement of CK and CK-MB or the cardiac specific troponins.

GAMMA-GLUTAMYL TRANSFERASE

PHYSIOLOGY AND BIOCHEMISTRY
Gamma-glutamyl transferase (GGT) is a microsomal enzyme responsible for the transfer of glutamyl groups from gamma-glutamyl peptides to other peptides or amino acids. It is present throughout the liver and hepatobiliary tree and in other organs such as the heart, kidneys, lungs, pancreas and seminal vesicles, although GGT activity in plasma is predominantly due to the liver isoenzyme. Plasma GGT is increased by enzyme inducing drugs such as phenytoin as well as alcohol.

USE IN CLINICAL PRACTICE
In patients with cholestasis, the plasma activity of GGT tends to change in parallel with alkaline phosphatase, but it is rather more sensitive to intra-hepatic cholestasis, which may help distinguish between patients with cirrhosis and cholangitis and guide subsequent investigations. When used in combination with

alkaline phosphatase a raised plasma GGT helps to confirm that any increase in alkaline phosphatase is of hepatic origin. GGT can also be useful in detecting alcohol misuse (Chapter 5).

ALKALINE PHOSPHATASE

PHYSIOLOGY AND BIOCHEMISTRY
The term alkaline phosphatase (ALP) is used to describe a group of enzymes which hydrolyse phosphate esters in alkaline solutions. Four structural genes encoding alkaline phosphatase have now been cloned and sequenced: a tissue non-specific ALP gene on chromosome 1 and genes for the intestinal, placental and germ cell ALP forms on chromosome 2. The last three genes and their products have considerable sequence homology (> 85%), whereas the tissue non-specific form has a sequence homology of only 50-60% compared with the other forms. As its name suggests, the tissue non-specific gene is widely expressed, being present in osteoblasts, hepatocytes and other cells. Tissue specific differences in the properties of the ALP from these various cells exists originating from differences in the carbohydrate side chains. The liver-derived isoenzyme is located on the exterior surface of the bile canalicular membrane and probably enters the bloodstream via the paracellular pathway (i.e., regurgitation from the canaliculus via the intracellullar junction complex and directly across the plasma membrane). In the circulation the plasma ALP activity is mainly derived from liver and bone isoenzymes with contributions from the intestinal form and from placental ALP during pregnancy.

USE IN CLINICAL PRACTICE
Plasma ALP activity rises in the presence of bile duct obstruction and this forms the basis of its clinical usefulness. The elevation is due neither to the failure of the liver to clear plasma ALP (as would be the case for bilirubin) nor to the release of ALP from damaged hepatocytes (as in the case of the aminotransferases). Rather, several pieces of evidence suggests that bile duct obstruction stimulates hepatic synthesis of ALP. In animal studies, no rise in plasma ALP occurs following bile duct obstruction if protein and RNA synthesis are blocked. Any obstruction to the bile duct may lead to an increase in plasma ALP activity. The obstruction may be at any level from high in the intrahepatic ducts (as in primary biliary cirrhosis) down to the common bile duct (due to gallstones, bile duct strictures or tumour). The rise in ALP may precede the onset of jaundice and, in those situations where relief of the obstruction is possible, plasma bilirubin concentration may return to normal before ALP.

As the methods for determining plasma ALP activity in use on routine biochemistry analysers measure total ALP, increases in the non-hepatic ALP isoenzymes will result in an elevated total ALP. This can be a problem in children where rapid bone growth results in an increase in the bone ALP isoenzyme, and in patients with bone disease or malignancy. This problem can be overcome by carrying out polyacrylamide gel electrophoresis on the plasma and staining specifically for ALP. Normally, three distinct bands will be seen on the gels corresponding to the liver, bone and intestinal ALP isoenzymes. An alternative approach is to repeat the standard ALP assay after heating the plasma sample at 56°C for 15 minutes. The liver and bone isoenzymes are sensitive to this treatment and, if the increased total ALP activity is due to either of them, it will be reduced to about 40% and 15% respectively of the original value. The placental isoenzyme remains unaffected by heat treatment. Obviously, this method is not as discriminatory as electrophoretic separation, but is easier to perform and can serve as a rough guide. An interesting, but uncommon, phenomenon is a transient hyperphosphatasaemia which occurs in children and very rarely in adults. The plasma total ALP rises sharply, often to 10-30 times the upper limit of normal, without evidence of acute liver or bone disease. Electrophoresis of plasma reveals a characteristic pattern of ALP isoenzymes with two bands that do not correspond to the normal liver and bone isoenzymes. These resolve into a single band following pre-treatment of plasma with neuraminidase suggesting that some alteration in sialylation of ALP occurs in this condition. In approximately 50% of cases transient hyperphosphatasaemia is associated with viral or bacterial infections, but it is itself benign and the plasma ALP normalizes over 3-6 weeks.

OTHER PLASMA ENZYMES

A number of other enzymes have been proposed over the years as possible replacements to ALP, GGT and the aminotransferases. 5'- Nucleotidase (5'-NT) which catalyses the hydrolysis of nucleotides and is located mainly on the canalicular membrane, was proposed as an improvement on ALP. 5'-NT rises in cholestatic conditions similar to those increasing ALP, but has the advantage of liver specificity, no increase being seen in bone disease. However, technical difficulties with the assay of 5'-NT have meant that, whilst occasionally used, it has not replaced ALP in routine biochemical liver profiles.

The glutathione S-transferase (GST) family of isoenzymes have emerged recently as potentially useful biochemical markers of liver disease now that plasma assays are available. The α-isoenzyme (GST-α) may become an alternative to the aminotransferases for assessing hepatocellular damage. Although found in low concentrations in the adrenals, testes and kidneys, the liver isoenzyme accounts for virtually all the GST-α activity in plasma. It has a half-life in blood of 90 minutes and provides a sensitive and rapidly responding marker of hepatocyte injury. Initial data suggests that GST-α is more sensitive than the aminotransferases for detection of drug-induced liver damage and may be superior to AST in identifying early rejection following liver transplantation. At present the ELISA format of the GST-α assay precludes its use in a routine setting but it may have a significant role in the future.

PLASMA PROTEINS

The liver is the site of synthesis of all plasma proteins except the immunoglobulins which are synthesized in the reticuloendothelial system. Figure 2.3 lists the most important plasma proteins made in the liver.

Plasma proteins secreted by the liver			
Protein	Molecular weight	Principle function	Plasma concentration (g/L)
Albumin	66,000	Binding and carrier protein, osmotic regulator	35 - 50
α1-antiprotease inhibitor	54,000	Elastase and trypsin inhibitor	1.0 - 2.0
α2-macroglobulin	720,000	General protease inhibitor	1.5 - 4.0
Antithrombin III	65,000	Protease inhibitor of coagulation system	0.15 - 0.3
Caeruloplasmin	134,000	Copper binding/transport	0.15 - 0.6
C-reactive protein	105,000	Opsonin	< 0.1
Fibrinogen	340,000	Fibrin precursor	2.0 - 4.5
Haptoglobin	100,000	Sequestration of free haemoglobin	0.8 - 1.8
Transferrin	80,000	Iron transport	2.0 - 4.0
Vitamin D binding protein	51,000	Vitamin D binding/transport	0.3 - 0.35

Figure 2.3 Plasma proteins secreted by the liver

Specific plasma proteins other than albumin which are important in the diagnosis of various liver disease are considered elsewhere including caeruloplasmin, transferrin and α1-antitrypsin (Chapter 4).

PLASMA ALBUMIN

BIOCHEMISTRY AND PHYSIOLOGY
Albumin is the major circulatory protein and is synthesized exclusively in the liver. About 12 g is synthesized each day and, of the total body pool of 300 g, about 60% is in the extravascular pool and 40% in the vascular pool. Albumin is unusual among proteins in that it has no carbohydrate side-chains, being a single polypeptide chain, 573 amino acids long. Prealbumin, the molecule synthesized on the rough endoplasmic reticulum (RER) has an additional 24 amino acid sequence which permits the nascent protein to be transferred across the RER. Removal of the first fifteen amino acids results in proalbumin which then migrates to the Golgi apparatus where cathepsin B removes the final five amino acids prior to secretion of albumin into the sinusoids. The half-life of albumin in the circulation is 21 days and the liver is probably the major site of breakdown. Albumin is responsible for maintaining plasma oncotic pressure and acts as a carrier protein binding numerous hormones, anions, drugs and fatty acids.

USE IN CLINICAL PRACTICE
Plasma albumin concentration is widely regarded as an index of hepatic 'synthetic function'. Whilst there is no doubt that chronic liver disease may indeed result in decreased albumin synthesis and consequent hypoalbuminaemia, several other important factors influence the plasma concentration and must be taken into account.

- The rate of hepatic albumin synthesis is governed by the availability of amino acids and falls sharply in protein malnutrition which may occur in alcoholic liver disease.
- Even when the rate of synthesis falls a compensatory reduction in the rate of degradation may maintain the plasma concentration for a period of time.
- Hypoalbuminaemia may be present with normal rates of synthesis when the protein leaks into the extravascular compartment as in ascites or when the plasma albumin is diluted by water retention.
- There is some evidence, particularly from animal studies, that alcohol may inhibit albumin secretion from hepatocytes, whilst synthesis proceeds normally.

When a patient presents with liver disease, the finding of a low plasma albumin is classically taken to indicate there is an underlying chronic component as the albumin half-life is long (21 days). Although as indicated above other factors than synthesis need to be considered in interpreting plasma albumin concentrations, hypoalbuminaemia is nearly always a poor prognostic feature in a liver disease patient.

PLASMA GLOBULINS
As part of the standard biochemical liver profile it is customary to estimate the total plasma globulin fraction as the difference between total protein and albumin. The immunoglobulins are discussed in detail elsewhere (Chapter 3). Any fall in plasma albumin tends to lead to a compensatory rise in the globulins, but extreme elevations (> 50 g/L) are usually only seen in autoimmune hepatitis and alcoholic liver disease.

PRACTICAL USE OF BIOCHEMICAL LIVER TESTS

In current practice the clinician wishing to assess liver function requests (or receives) a panel of several test results. The pattern of abnormality provides additional information to that provided by the individual tests. Thus having described these individual tests in some detail the practical aspects of recognising characteristic patterns of results in different clinical situations is now considered. It is not uncommon for textbooks to give tables or diagrams of the numerical values of 'LFT's' in different diagnostic categories. This is misleading: in any condition the tests are not static but change with time and treatment. It is more useful to consider the tests in certain distinct clinical situations:

- at initial presentation when the pattern of results may help determine the type of liver disease present i.e., hepatocellular versus cholestatic,
- monitoring progression of established disease or the response to treatment,
- as prognostic indicators,
- in circumstances where abnormal results have been obtained in a patient in whom hepatic disease was not suspected - the tests having been undertaken as a screening procedure.

BIOCHEMICAL LIVER TESTS IN HEPATOCELLULAR AND CHOLESTATIC LIVER DISEASE
The principle cause of hepatocellular injury are those conditions characterised by inflammation: viral, autoimmune or drug induced hepatitis. Cholestasis may be either intra- or extra hepatic (Chapter 1). In cholestasis there is a tendency for all substances secreted in the bile to accumulate in the plasma, although bilirubin may not always rise in the early stages of the disease. Other characteristic biochemical features are bilirubinuria (even in the absence of jaundice) and elevation of plasma ALP and GGT activities to a greater degree than the aminotransferases. Plasma cholesterol, triglycerides and bile acids may also increase

markedly. In contrast, in the acute phase of hepatocellular liver disease the amino-transferases are markedly increased with normal or near normal plasma ALP and GGT activities. Thus, by considering the relative activities of the plasma enzymes it is possible to gain some idea as to whether the liver disease has a cholestatic or hepatocellular origin. It is important to remember that these tests are not in themselves diagnostic but serve as a guide to the most appropriate second stage of investigations e.g., serology, imaging, etc. The changes in the standard biochemical liver tests in individual disease states are considered in later chapters.

BIOCHEMICAL LIVER TESTS FOR MONITORING RESPONSE TO THERAPY

Liver biopsy and sophisticated imaging tests may be very helpful in establishing a diagnosis but thereafter they are not suitable for frequent repetition to assess progress, both in view of cost and safety aspects, and it is here that the standard biochemical liver tests find their greatest use.

The plasma aminotransferases can be used to monitor the response to immuno-suppressive therapy in patients with autoimmune hepatitis. Once treatment is commenced plasma AST and bilirubin should fall to normal within a few weeks if remission is induced. Any subsequent rise in AST to over three times the upper reference interval is consistently associated with histological and clinical relapse and the AST rise usually antedates symptoms permitting dosage adjustments to be made. Similarly, after surgical treatment of biliary obstruction or resection of tumours the plasma bilirubin and ALP can be helpful in assessing the success of the treatment and as an aid to early recognition of complications. The standard biochemical liver tests are particularly valuable in monitoring patients following liver transplantation: this is discussed in greater detail in Chapter 9.

BIOCHEMICAL LIVER TESTS AS INDICATORS OF PROGNOSIS

A low plasma albumin, impaired clotting and raised bilirubin are features associated with poor prognosis in patients with chronic liver disease, but the confidence limits are usually so wide that in the individual patient little significance can be attached. However, in certain circumstances more precise figures have been obtained and various scoring systems proposed which incorporate clinical, biochemical and haematological parameters (Figure 2.4). Scoring systems have also been derived for acute hepatic failure, particularly following paracetamol overdosage, which can be helpful in selecting patients for urgent liver transplantation. (Figure 2.5).

Scoring systems for liver disease	
CHILD-PUGH SCORE FOR CIRRHOSIS Ascites (extent) Encephalopathy (grade) Plasma albumin Plasma bilirubin	MAYO CLINIC PBC SCORE Plasma albumin Plasma bilirubin INR Age Oedema (extent and response to diuretics)
MAYO CLINIC PSC SCORE Haemoglobin Plasma bilirubin Inflammatory bowel disease Histological stage Age	KINGS PSC SCORE Hepatomegaly Splenomegaly Histological stage Plasma alkaline phosphatase Age

Figure 2.4 Scoring systems for predicting prognosis in liver disease

Scoring system for paracetamol overdosage
· INR (rising on day 4 after overdosage)
· Arterial hydrogen ion concentration > 50 nmol/L
· INR > 7.0
· Plasma creatinine > 300 µmol/L
· Grade III/IV encephalopathy

Figure 2.5 King's College Hospital scoring system for predicting poor prognosis following paracetamol overdosage

ABNORMAL LFTS IN THE ABSENCE OF SYMPTOMS OF LIVER DISEASE

Up to 50% of patients with chronic liver disease will already have progressed to cirrhosis before they first present with any signs or symptoms of liver disease, while other patients with cirrhosis may have no symptoms unless malignant change develops. Furthermore, cirrhosis is not uncommonly found incidentally at autopsy. Thus it is clear that there must be a considerable amount of subclinical liver disease in the population and it is not surprising that, with the use of test requesting profiles and health screening programmes which provide the physician with biochemical liver tests routinely, abnormalities are found in patients without overt signs and symptoms.

Alcohol misuse is the commonest factor implicated. The finding of a raised GGT and/or AST is usually associated with fatty liver related to obesity, often in association with diabetes or excess alcohol consumption. Less common causes include asymptomatic chronic hepatitis and haemochromatosis. Although further tests may help in narrowing the differential diagnosis, ultimately histological examination of the liver biopsy may be required for a definitive diagnosis. Bearing in mind the previously mentioned physiological and non-hepatic pathological causes, isolated increases of ALP activity are otherwise usually attributable to subclinical primary biliary cirrhosis or metastatic tumours. Asymptomatic hyperbilirubinaemia is most likely to be due to Gilbert's syndrome, but haemolytic diseases e.g., sickle cell disease or congenital spherocytosis must be considered.

OTHER BIOCHEMICAL TESTS FOR LIVER DISEASE

Other biochemical tests specific for particular disease are discussed in the appropriate chapters of this book. There are, however, two classes of tests which have more general applications, tests of hepatic fibrosis and the quantitative liver function tests.

TESTS OF HEPATIC FIBROSIS

Measurement of fibrosis, which is a characteristic feature of chronic liver disease and responsible for several of the complications thereof, would assist in monitoring the progression of disease and may allow optimisation of therapy. The only accurate assessment of the degree of fibrosis is histological examination of the liver tissue, but for the purpose of monitoring disease repeat liver biopsies is undesirable. A number of candidate markers have been measured in plasma (Figure 2.6), but the only marker that has found routine application has been the aminoterminal procollagen type III peptide (PIIINP).

As liver disease progresses control of collagen synthesis becomes deranged and increased collagen deposition occurs. Procollagen peptides are globular proteins which are cleaved from the ends of the procollagen molecule by procollagen endopeptidases. Many studies have now been carried out on the use of PIIINP in liver disease and it appears the plasma PIIINP concentration reflects fibrinogenesis (i.e., the rate of ongoing fibrosis) rather than the absolute amount of fibrosis present in the liver. PIIINP measurements have found a use in the monitoring of patients on chronic methotrexate therapy where hepatic fibrosis can occur (Chapter 5).

Markers for hepatic fibrosis
• Procollagen III peptide aminoterminal (PIIINP)
• Prolyl hydroxylase
• Laminin
• Fibronectin
• Type 7S collagen

Figure 2.6 Candidate biochemical markers in plasma for hepatic fibrosis

TESTS OF HEPATOCELLULAR ACTIVITY (QUANTITATIVE LIVER
FUNCTION TESTS)

With the exception of albumin (synthetic function) and bilirubin (conjugation and excretion) most of the biochemical liver tests described in this chapter are indicators of liver damage rather than function. Ideally, quantitative assessment of the functional hepatic mass would allow the hepatologist to judge when patients with acute or chronic liver disease were nearing end-stage hepatic failure and plan therapeutic interventions such as liver transplantation accordingly. Various tests have been proposed based on the ability of the liver to clear exogenous compounds from the body (Figure 2.7).

Quantitative tests for hepatocellular activity
• Galactose elimination capacity
• Aminopyrine breath test
• Indocyanine green clearance
• Monoethylglycineexylidide formation test

Figure 2.7 Quantitative tests of hepatocellular activity

The galactose elimination capacity (GEC) measures the zero-order clearance of intravenously administered galactose by hepatic phosphorylation. It has been used to predict survival in patients with late stage primary biliary cirrhosis and to monitor interferon therapy in chronic viral hepatitis. The aminopyrine breath test (APBT) is based on the cytochrome (CYP) P450 dependent demethylation of isotopically labelled (^{13}C or ^{14}C) aminopyrine to carbon dioxide. The test has been used in similar circumstances to the galactose elimination capacity. Indocyanine green clearance has been reported to be superior to both GEC and APBT for discriminating disease severity in cirrhotic patients, possibly because it incorporates a measure of liver blood flow in its assessment of hepatocellular function. This may serve as a measure of the presence and extent of portal hypertension and oesophageal varices present in chronic liver disease patients. The monoethyl-glycinexylidide formation test (MEGX), like APBT, is also a CYP450-dependent test based on hepatic metabolism of intravenously administered lignocaine to MEGX. As the test only requires measurement (automated) of MEGX in a single blood sample taken 15-30 minutes after a bolus of lignocaine, the test has been studied in many different groups of patients, with varying degrees of success. Older clearance tests, such as caffeine clearance and the bromsulphthalein test, are now only of historical interest. As clearance tests, in the main, require specialist measuring techniques their use is predominantly confined to specialist liver units.

A further test of hepatocellular function is the arterial ketone body ratio (AKBR), which is the ratio of acetoacetate to 3-hydroxybutyrate in arterial blood. The AKBR reflects hepatic mitochondrial function and redox state. Reductions in AKBR are associated with poor prognosis in patients following hepatic surgery or in fulminant hepatic failure.

HAEMATOLOGICAL TESTS IN LIVER FUNCTION

INTRODUCTION
The liver plays a central role in the maintenance of normal haematopoesis and haemostasis. Whilst in adults the bone marrow is primarily responsible for the production of red cells, platelets and granulocytes, subsequent red cell breakdown and bilirubin metabolism occur principally in the liver. In early fetal life, however, the liver is also the site of haematopoesis and may become so again in adult life when bone marrow function is compromised. Most of the coagulation factors and their inhibitors are synthesised in the liver, as are the circulatory binding proteins for iron and vitamin B12, which, together with folic acid, are all stored in the liver.

To this extent it is predictable that liver disease will lead to haematological problems including disturbances of haemostasis and abnormal numbers and function of the formed elements of blood. In addition, however, in liver disease there are inhibitors of chemotaxis and neutrophil abnormalities. These may lead to an increased susceptibility to bacterial infection, which is not directly related to disturbances of the known haematological functions of the liver.

ABNORMALITIES OF HAEMOSTASIS

Patients with liver disease are prone to bruising, bleeding after venipuncture and nose bleeds. In liver failure, spontaneous haemorrhage into vital structures may occur, and variceal haemorrhage may be difficult to arrest when coagulation factors are deficient. Despite the fact that bleeding problems are only occasionally severe, assessment of the clotting factors may be useful as indicators of liver function, and as a guide to the likelihood of bleeding after invasive procedures such as percutaneous liver biopsy.

PHYSIOLOGY AND BIOCHEMISTRY

The mechanism by which blood clots only at the appropriate place and time, and the consequent lysis of the clot, are extremely complex. Only those aspects relevant to the tests used in liver disease are considered in any detail in this chapter and readers are referred to appropriate haematological texts if further detail is required.

Damage to blood vessels sets in motion a complex sequence of enzymatic reactions which convert inactive circulating molecules into active forms which finally results in the formation of a clot consisting of a fibrin framework and platelets. This cascade (Figure 2.8) is initiated either by contact of the blood with subendothelial collagen (the intrinsic pathway) or by the release of thromboplastin (the extrinsic pathway) at the site of the vascular damage. Both these pathways lead ultimately (via the common pathway) to the conversion of prothrombin to thrombin which, in turn, converts fibrinogen to fibrin. The coagulation cascade is controlled by inhibitory factors, and by clearance of activated coagulation factors by the liver. Clots are broken down by the fibrinolytic system (Figure 2.9).

Plasminogen is activated by several factors to form plasmin which digests fibrin leading to the formation of fibrin degradation products (FDPs). Plasmin, together with α2-macroglobulin, protein C and antithrombin III (ATIII) are natural inhibitors of coagulation. ATIII is the most powerful inhibitor and is present in decreased concentrations in patients with liver disease.

TESTS OF COAGULATION

As part of the investigation of liver disease it is possible to measure the concentrations of the individual clotting factors. More often, tests, such as the prothrombin time, which measure the cumulative effect of a number of factors at the same time are used.

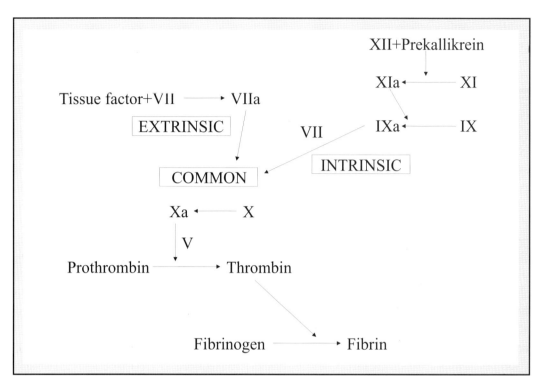

Figure 2.8 The clotting cascade

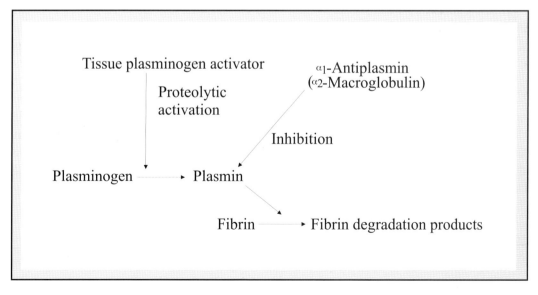

Figure 2.9 The fibrinolytic system

The one-stage prothrombin time (PT) test measures the rate at which prothrombin is converted to thrombin in the presence of activated clotting factors, calcium and thromboplastin. The PT will screen for deficiencies in the factors involved in the extrinsic and common pathways, i.e., factors VII, V and X, prothrombin and fibrinogen. The normal PT is between 12 and 16 seconds, although each time the test is performed a normal control is included and the result expressed as a ratio (International Normalised Ratio (INR)) of the patient's time to the normal control, or in 'seconds prolonged' again in relation to the normal control. Prolongation of the PT by more than 3 seconds (or INR > 1.2) is usually considered abnormal. A raised INR is a contra-indication to carrying out a liver biopsy. Measurement of clotting times is incorporated in many scoring systems used to grade disease severity in both chronic and acute liver disease (see Chapter 1, Figure 1.9). In patients with acute hepatic failure an INR greater than 7.0 is a poor prognostic feature and is one of the criteria for listing a patient for emergency liver trans-plantation.

If the plasma fibrinogen concentration is normal (> 5 g/L), then a prolonged PT suggests a deficiency of one of the four factors involved or of vitamin K. Four of these coagulation factors, prothrombin (II), VII, IX and X are synthesised in the liver in precursor form and have no coagulation activity until modified by vitamin K. Vitamin K is required for the carboxylation of the terminal glutamic acid residues of these factors prior to glycosylation and secretion. Hypovitaminosis K thus results in prolongation of the PT. Specific congenital deficiencies exist (e.g., Christmas disease, where factor IX is deficient), but in most cases of liver disease the deficiency is acquired. Severe protein malnutrition will also cause deficiencies of clotting factors. Vitamin K is present in most vegetables (K1) and is also formed in the gut by bacteria (K2). Being a fat soluble vitamin, effective absorption of dietary vitamin K from the gut requires bile salts and thus where there is cholestasis, vitamin K concentrations fall rapidly because body stores are small.

If an abnormal PT 'corrects' after parenteral administration of vitamin K, it may be assumed that the defect was due to vitamin K deficiency, and, providing dietary deficiency can be excluded, inferred that some cholestasis was present. On the other hand, if the abnormal PT persists after vitamin K administration, then deficiency of one or more of the coagulation factors due to poor hepatic synthetic function may be assumed. In practice, 10 mg of vitamin K is given parenterally and the PT measured again 24 h later. If the PT returns to normal, or improves by at least 50%, then hypovitaminosis K and some degree of cholestasis may be assumed.

DISSEMINATED INTRAVASCULAR COAGULATION

Disseminated intravascular coagulation (DIC) is a haemorrhagic syndrome in which initiation of the coagulation cascade leads to widespread intravascular coagulation, 'consumption' of circulating coagulation factors and platelets and a consequent fibrinolytic process. It is characterised by a low platelet count, damaged red cells (schistocytes), low fibrinogen concentration, prolonged PT and high titres of fibrinogen degradation products (FDPs). The thrombin time is prolonged if the fibrinogen concentration is low or FDPs are present, but if these are normal an acquired dysfibrinogenaemia should be suspected (abnormal fibrinogen molecules with increased sialic acid content in their carbohydrate side chains). The diagnosis of DIC in patients with liver disease is difficult because the abnormalities listed above can be present for reasons other than DIC and many patients have a chronic low grade DIC of no clinical significance.

ANAEMIA AND ABNORMALITIES OF THE RED BLOOD CELLS

Anaemia is common in patients with liver disease and its cause is multi factorial. However, to some degree the 'anaemia', as measured by the haemoglobin concentration or packed cell volume (PCV), may be apparent rather than real because blood volume is often increased in patients with cirrhosis. In addition, there is the normochromic normocytic anaemia which can be seen in any chronic disease.

IRON DEFICIENCY ANAEMIA

Microcytic anaemia is seen in patients who are losing blood and may be compounded by inadequate dietary iron intake. The site of blood loss is usually the gut, either from oesophageal varices or peptic ulceration, both of which frequently complicate chronic liver disease. There may be malaena or fresh blood in the stool, but faecal occult blood testing may be required for its detection.

MACROCYTOSIS AND MEGALOBLASTIC ANAEMIA

An elevated mean corpuscular volume (MCV) and macrocytes evident on the blood film are very common in patients with liver disease and/or misusing alcohol. Two distinct causes need to be distinguished: first, idiopathic 'macrocytosis of alcoholic liver disease' which is the most common cause (up to 60%) and second, megaloblastic anaemia due to dietary folate deficiency. Idiopathic macrocytosis may be a consequence of abnormal profiles of lipids in the circulation which alter the structure of the red cell membrane, or a prolonged cell-cycle time during which the cell continues to grow. The macrocytes are thin (leptocytes) and although the MCV is high (100 - 150 fL), the mean corpuscular haemoglobin concentration is normal. There is no associated anaemia and plasma and red cell folate and vitamin B12 concentrations are normal. Macrocytosis is also a side effect of treatment with azothiaprine which is used in the treatment of autoimmune hepatitis and following liver transplantation.

In alcoholic patients, however, dietary deficiency of folate is common and macrocytosis with associated megaloblastic anaemia often develops over time. Associated findings are hypersegmented neutrophils, a mild unconjugated hyperbilirubinaemia and megaloblastic myeloid and erythroid precursors in the bone marrow. Red cell folate is a more sensitive measure of folate deficiency than plasma folate. Vitamin B12 concentrations are usually normal but pernicious anaemia may co-exist and it is always important to measure plasma B12 in patients with megaloblastic changes. After prolonged folate deficiency, sideroblastic changes develop with a hypochromic anaemia despite normal or elevated plasma iron and transferrin saturation.

HAEMOLYTIC ANAEMIA

This is an occasional complication in patients with primary biliary cirrhosis, autoimmune hepatitis and in alcoholic patients with Zieve's syndrome. The latter comprises acute haemolysis, unconjugated jaundice and increased plasma lipids occurring in a patient with alcohol-related liver disease. Many patients with chronic liver disease have a low-grade chronic haemolysis which is of little clinical significance. Reticulocytosis often occurs after stopping heavy alcohol consumption and does not necessarily imply haemolysis.

APLASTIC ANAEMIA

Aplastic anaemia is a very rare, but potentially fatal, complication of acute viral hepatitis. Patients receiving azothiaprine may also become aplastic if the dose is not monitored carefully and altered appropriately taking into account genetic polymorphism in azothiaprine metabolism (Chapter 5).

HYPERSPLENISM.

Patients with chronic liver disease often have enlarged spleens and this is invariably associated with some degree of pancytopaenia: the platelet and granulocyte counts are particularly low. The mechanism is not fully understood, but is probably a combination of sequestration of blood cells, increased plasma volume and some degree of haemolysis. It is not uncommon to see platelet counts well below 50×10^9/L, a level which, under other circumstances, is associated with a risk of spontaneous haemorrhage. However, in patients with hypersplenism this type of pancytopaenia is usually benign and although splenectomy may be effective in 'improving' the blood count, the operative risk usually outweighs any benefit to the patient.

ABNORMALITIES OF WHITE BLOOD CELLS

The high risk of bacterial infection in patients with chronic liver disease is related to disturbances in function rather than in the number of granulocytes, except following treatment with azothiaprine or cytotoxic agents. There are defects in opsonization (the process whereby micro-organisms are coated with immunoglobulins and/or complement so as to be recognised by neutrophils as foreign), and plasma factors inhibit chemoattractant activity. In acute liver disease, particularly acute hepatic failure, decreased complement concentrations may account for the high frequency of bacterial infection. Atypical lymphocytes are not uncommon in patients with acute viral hepatitis.

FURTHER READING.

Bowman BH. Hepatic Plasma Proteins; Mechanism of Function and Regulation. Academic Press, San Diego 1993.

Johnson PJ. Role of the standard 'liver function tests' in current clinical practice. Ann Clin Biochem. 1989; **25:** 463-71.

Kelly DA, Tuddenham ECG. Haemostatic problems in liver disease. Gut 1986; **27:** 339-49.

Lindenbaum J. Haematologic complications in alcohol abuse. Sem Liver Dis 1987; **3:** 169-81.

Moss DM. Perspectives in alkaline phosphatase research. Clin Chem. 1992; **38:** 2486-92.

Sallie R, Tredger JM, Williams R. Drugs and the liver. Part 1:Testing liver function. Biopharm Drugs Dispos 1991; **12:** 251-9.

Tredger JM, Sherwood RA. The liver; new functional, prognostic and diagnostic tests. Ann Clin Biochem 1997; **34:** 121-41.

Chapter 3

Infectious liver disease

INTRODUCTION

Many infectious agents are capable of causing liver disease in humans, but the most important epidemiologically are viral, trematode and cestode infections. Viral infections are the commonest cause of acute hepatitis. The range of responsible viruses is very broad but those of greatest importance are the hepatitis viruses A, B, C, D and E. The viral hepatitis 'alphabet' is still growing. It has been suggested that there may be an F virus, although this has not been confirmed, and a hepatitis G virus (designated GBV-C/HGV) has been identified but recent evidence indicates that it only rarely causes significant liver damage. Trematode and cestode infections of the liver are exceedingly common in tropical and some sub-tropical areas. They are less prevalent in temperate zones but infections may remain dormant for many years and are therefore not uncommon among immigrant communities in non-endemic areas. Diagnosis can be difficult because there may be concurrent infections with the hepatitis viruses, which are endemic in the same areas where these worm infections are prevalent.

VIRAL HEPATITIS

The hepatitis viruses are distinguished from each other by their morphology, modes of transmission and propensity for development of chronic infections (Figure 3.1). The A and E viruses are transmitted via the faecal-oral route and cause acute hepatitis with very rarely any long-term sequelae, while the B, C and D viruses are parenterally-transmitted and are associated with development of chronic hepatitis following the initial acute phase. The true incidence of acute and chronic viral hepatitis throughout the world is unknown because it is often not diagnosed, but the World Health Organisation estimates that there are about 350 million chronic carriers of hepatitis B virus worldwide and at least 300 million people who are chronically infected with hepatitis C virus. With all of these viruses, the highest prevalence is among the peoples of Asia, Africa, South America, and Eastern, Central and Southern Europe. However, hepatitis A and C viruses are also common in Western Europe and North America, where there are also pockets of endemic hepatitis B virus infection (mainly among the sexually promiscuous and intravenous drug users).

The sequence of events following infections with these viruses varies widely and depends on which virus is involved, how and at what age the infection is acquired, the viral load in the inoculum and the host's response to it. In all instances, after a period of incubation (which varies between the different viruses from 2 to 26 weeks) there is an acute phase. This typically begins with general malaise, nausea and loss of appetite, with fatigue and often abdominal pain or discomfort and an influenza-like illness (fever, myalgia and arthralgia), followed by the appearance of dark urine and pale faeces and the development of jaundice. However, this phase is often entirely asymptomatic. Conversely, it can occasionally follow a particularly severe course which may progress to acute liver failure (Chapter 1) and coma, with a high mortality. In most cases, the acute phase gradually resolves over a period of several weeks or months. The outcome then depends on which virus is involved. As noted above, there are usually no long-term sequelae with the hepatitis A and E viruses but the B, C and D viruses can lead to chronic liver disease of varying severity. The mechanisms of liver damage in acute or chronic hepatitis virus infections are not fully understood. The available evidence suggests that the viruses are not overtly cytopathic and that hepatocellular injury is probably due to host immune reactions against virus-infected cells but, at least in hepatitis A and B infections, virus-induced autoimmune reactions may also play a role (see Chapter 6).

The hepatitis viruses					
	Virus				
	A	**B**	**C**	**D**	**E**
Genome	RNA	DNA	RNA	RNA	RNA
Taxonomy	'Hepatovirus'	Hepadnavirus	Flavivirus	Unclassified (similarities with plant viriods)	Hepevirus
Transmission	Faecal/oral	Parenteral	Parenteral	Parenteral	Parenteral
Chronic infection	No	Yes	Yes	Yes	No

Figure 3.1 Comparison of some of the features of the different hepatitis viruses

The plasma biochemical changes reflect pathological processes which are similar for all hepatitis virus infections. During the early acute phase (even before the development of symptoms), plasma aminotransferases begin to rise and may reach concentrations more than 50 times the reference limits. In contrast to alcoholic hepatitis (Chapter 5), plasma alanine aminotransferase (ALT) is usually higher than aspartate aminotransferase (AST). As the acute illness subsides, ALT and AST activities return to normal (although they may continue to be moderately elevated for several weeks or months in protracted cases or in chronic infections). Plasma bilirubin concentrations rise more slowly, eventually peaking at 10-20 times the reference limit, but alkaline phosphatase (ALP) and γ-glutamyl transferase (GGT) activities are generally only mildly elevated. Mild to moderate hyperglobulinaemia (mainly IgM and IgG) is a frequent finding and various autoantibodies may become detectable (see Chapter 6).

HEPATITIS A

The hepatitis A virus (HAV) is a 27 nm RNA virus which was originally included within the genus Enterovirus but has since been classified as a prototype virus of the new genus 'hepatovirus'. The usual mode of transmission via the faecal-oral route occurs mainly through personal contact (especially among children), the drinking of contaminated water or the consumption of shellfish (particularly filter feeders that concentrate the virus, such as clams and other bivalves) harvested from sewage-contaminated waters. However, in recent years improvements in hygienic conditions (especially through better sanitation and control of food handling, water supplies and sewage treatment) and vaccination programmes have led to dramatic reductions in HAV infections in countries with low or intermediate endemicity. The clinical course is often benign and patients may not even know they have been infected. Occasionally, it may present as a severe cholestatic illness or (rarely) develop into acute liver failure (Chapter 1) but overall the prognosis is excellent. There are reports of protracted infections with HAV relapsing over several months but true chronic infections seem not to occur.

HAV SEROLOGY

After infection, the virus replicates in the liver during the incubation period. A low-grade viraemia develops, reaching a peak just before the onset of symptoms and disappearing rapidly as the clinical illness commences (Figure 3.2). During this time, virus particles are shed in the stools and the patient is highly infectious. The onset of symptoms coincides with the development of a primary antibody (IgM anti-HAV) response to the virus, which continues with rising titres during the acute phase (Figure 3.2). During recovery, titres of IgM anti-HAV usually fall and patients become seronegative but sometimes the IgM anti-HAV persists at a lower level, which may reflect prolonged acute (and, therefore, potentially still infectious) disease.

Shortly after the onset of symptoms, the secondary (IgG) antibody response begins and titres of IgG anti-HAV continue to rise for several months after recovery.

Thereafter, they may decline to a lower level, but subjects usually remain seropositive for life and this antibody appears to provide protection against re-infection. During the viraemic phase, HAV-specific antigen and viral genomic material (HAV-RNA) can be detected in the plasma and stools. However, these markers disappear rapidly with the onset of symptoms and are often missed, and the techniques required for their detection do not readily lend themselves to routine screening. Thus the diagnostic serology for HAV infection is the finding of IgM anti-HAV in the plasma, with IgG antibody being a reflection of past infection.

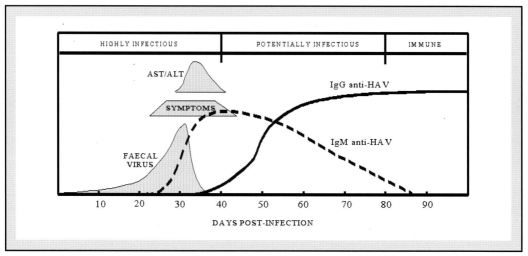

Figure 3.2 Serological events in hepatitis A virus (HAV) infection

HEPATITIS B

The hepatitis B virus (HBV) is one of a group of Hepadna viruses that infect man and other animals. Horizontal transmission used to occur mainly during blood transfusions or injection of blood products but, in most countries, screening for HBV in blood donors and the development of vaccination programmes have led to a marked reduction in the number of infections acquired in this way, while careful monitoring of HBV-positive mothers and therapeutic intervention in the newborn is beginning to reduce vertical (maternal/fetal) transmission in many of the industrialised nations. In these countries, infection is now largely confined to certain high-risk groups, e.g., intravenous drug users and the sexually promiscuous. Elsewhere, vertical transmission is probably the most important factor in maintaining the high level of infection in the population, because neonates who acquire the virus almost always become chronic carriers.

Worldwide about 5% of adults infected with HBV fail to clear the virus within six months. Most of these will remain chronically infected but about 1% per year spontaneously clear the virus. In contrast, 95% of babies infected perinatally become chronically infected and very rarely clear the virus during their lifetime. Chronic infection is associated with several possible outcomes. Many individuals are asymptomatic and, indeed, used to be designated 'healthy carriers'. However, it is now known that most have at least some morphological changes in their livers. In some, the changes will be relatively mild and may not progress. Others will have florid liver damage that rapidly progresses to cirrhosis, even if they lack clinical symptoms in the early stages. About 5% of patients with cirrhosis due to chronic hepatitis B develop hepatocellular carcinoma each year, but it is not clear whether this is because HBV is inherently oncogenic or whether it is related to the cirrhosis, which itself is known to predispose to malignancy (Chapter 7).

HBV SEROLOGY

The complete HBV virion is a 42 nm particle with a circular DNA core surrounded by a protein coat (Figure 3.3). The virus carries its own specific DNA polymerase and a primase. Electron microscopic examination of plasma obtained during an acute infection reveals numerous particles of different sizes. In addition to the 42 nm particle, there are 22 nm spheres and filamentous structures of variable length which together vastly outnumber the full virus particles. These represent excess coat protein which the virus produces in copious amounts. This was the first plasma marker of HBV infection to be identified and was formerly known as 'Australia antigen' (it was initially discovered in the blood of an Australian aborigine), but it is now termed hepatitis B surface antigen (HBsAg). The viral DNA is encapsulated within a second protein, the core protein (HBc). This is not normally detected in plasma because it is usually enclosed within the surface antigen coat and, in any event, any exposed HBc will be complexed with its specific antibody (anti-HBc) which blocks its detection. However, a closely related

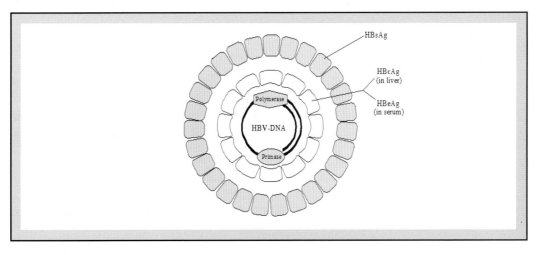

Figure 3.3 Schematic representation of the hepatitis B virus (HBV)

protein, the 'e' antigen (HBeAg), which is thought to be derived from HBc by proteolytic cleavage, can be detected in plasma and is almost always associated with the presence of the complete virion.

Infection with HBV is followed by development of marked viraemia during the prodromal phase, reaching a peak shortly before the development of symptoms. This can be demonstrated by the finding of HBsAg and HBeAg, as well HBV-DNA in plasma (Figure 3.4). At or about the onset of symptoms, the virus elicits a primary (IgM) antibody response to the core protein and the IgM anti-HBc titre rises as the illness progresses. Disappearance of full virus particles from the blood begins during the acute phase, usually before the peak in plasma aminotransferase activities, and patients typically become HBeAg negative as symptoms subside. During this period, however, large quantities of the coat protein (HBsAg) continue to be produced by the infected liver and HBsAg may persist in the blood for several weeks after recovery, before gradually disappearing. As the viraemia wanes, antibodies to the 'e' antigen (anti-HBe) begin to appear in the plasma and their titre may continue to rise for several months (Figure 3.4). This switch from HBe antigenaemia to anti-HBe production is known as seroconversion and it heralds a period during which the patient becomes progressively less infectious. Complete confidence that the individual is no longer infectious comes, however, only with the disappearance of HBsAg and a second seroconversion with appearance of anti-HBs antibodies. This is accompanied by a gradual reduction of IgM anti-HBc and rising titres of IgG class anti-HBc, which reach a plateau and then usually persist at lower levels for life (affording protection against re-infection).

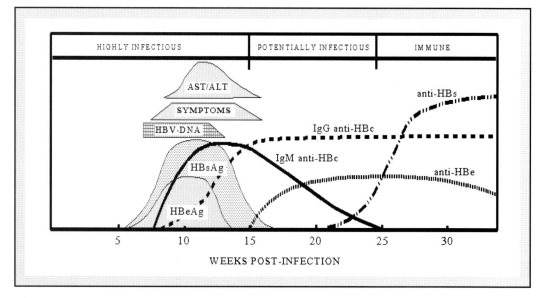

Figure 3.4 Typical sequence of serological events in acute HBV infection

Screening for HBV infection involves testing for HBsAg in plasma. Seropositive individuals are then usually tested for HBeAg and anti-HBe, and often for IgM anti-HBc, to determine the status of their infection. Progress of the infection is usually monitored by testing for the development of anti-HBe and anti-HBs and the gradual disappearance of IgM anti-HBc. Testing for HBV-DNA is still quite costly and is usually performed only when it is necessary to confirm the diagnosis in patients with atypical infections or for monitoring the disappearance of the virus during antiviral therapy.

SEROLOGY OF CHRONIC HBV INFECTION
The initial clinical and biochemical features in individuals who develop chronic hepatitis B depend on how and when the infection is acquired but are often mild or even sub-clinical, and may be missed if jaundice does not develop. At unpredictable intervals after the acute phase aminotransferases may become normal but HBsAg, HBeAg and IgM anti-HBc persist and patients remain highly infectious (Figure 3.5). This phase may last for life but many patients will eventually seroconvert, either spontaneously or in response to antiviral therapy. This is usually associated with what appears to be a second episode of acute hepatitis, with a 'flare' of aminotransferase activity accompanied by the disappearance of HBeAg and IgM anti-HBc and the development of anti-HBe (Figure 3.5).

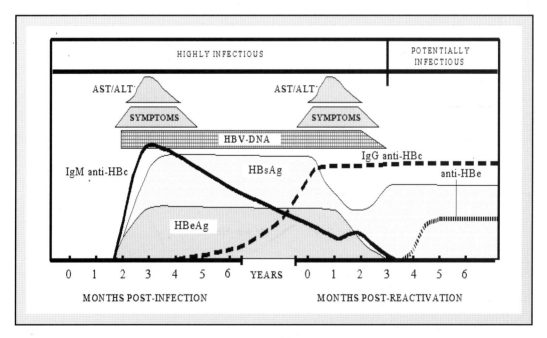

Figure 3.5 Typical sequence of serological events in chronic hepatitis B following an acute infection. Note: seroconversion from HBeAg to anti-HBe may occur after many months or (as shown) years, but HBeAg may persist for life

Seropositivity for HBsAg usually persists but this may also eventually disappear, and patients may become anti-HBs positive. However, recent evidence indicates that such individuals may continue to be HBV-DNA seropositive at low titre and may harbour the virus in their livers or peripheral blood mononuclear cells for long periods. They therefore remain potentially infectious.

ATYPICAL HBV SEROLOGY

Occasionally, patients with HBV infection are found to be seronegative for HBsAg and HBeAg on routine testing during the acute phase. This situation can arise when the viraemia is short-lived and peaks before the onset of symptoms. Often, the clinical impression can be confirmed by demonstrating anti-HBe and/or anti-HBs in the plasma. Occasionally, however, the antibody responses are slow to develop and the patient may be found to be seronegative for all four of these markers (HBsAg, HBeAg, anti-HBe and anti-HBs) for a time. This period is known as the 'core window' and the only serological evidence of the infection will be the presence of IgM anti-HBc (Figure 3.6).

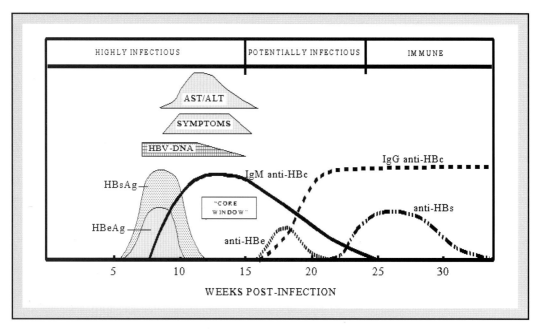

Figure 3.6 Atypical serology in acute hepatitis B. Note the so-called 'core window' during which IgM anti-HBc may be the only marker detected

Additionally, it is now known that the virus has the ability to mutate under host immune pressure and thereby avoid detection by the host's immune system. The frequency with which this process of 'escape mutation' occurs is unknown, but there are now several examples of mutations leading to alterations in the core, 'e' and surface antigens. A comprehensive discussion is beyond the scope of this book. Suffice it to say that, when such mutations occur, the infected subject may show serological markers of seroconversion, with apparent elimination of the virus, only to continue to be infected by the mutant form.

HEPATITIS C

The hepatitis C virus (HCV) was identified in 1989 as the major agent responsible for what, until then, had been termed non-A, non-B viral hepatitis. It is a positive-stranded RNA virus which is related to the agents that cause a number of arthropod-borne viral diseases including yellow fever and Dengue fever, and to the pestiviruses that infect animals, and it has been classified as a separate genus within the family Flaviviridae. It is transmitted parenterally, but in about 50% of cases no history of parenteral exposure to blood or blood products is obtained. The route of transmission in these so-called 'community-acquired' infections remains unknown. The virus has a worldwide distribution but its prevalence in the general population varies from less than 0.2% in north-east England to more than 10% in some parts of North Africa.

The HCV genome is approximately 9.6 kb in length, with short untranslated regions at the 5' and 3' ends and a single open reading frame that encodes a polyprotein of about 3000 amino acid residues (Figure 3.7). The latter is processed by a combination of viral and host proteases to yield a number of structural and non-structural components.

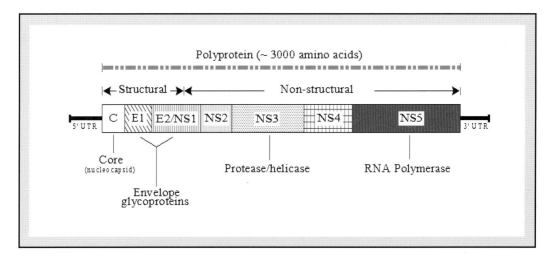

Figure 3.7 Schematic representation of the hepatitis C virus (HCV) genome

The structural components include a core protein (C) that encapsidates the genomic RNA and two glycoproteins (E1 and E2) that are presumed to be integrated in the viral envelope. The non-structural components include the viral proteases as well as a helicase and an RNA-polymerase that are thought to be involved in replication of the virus. Phylogenetic analyses have identified six main genotypes (1 to 6) of the virus, each with a number of sub-types (designated a, b, c, etc.), which vary in their geographical distribution around the world and in the severity of the liver disease that they cause.

In contrast to HBV, up to 80% of adults exposed to HCV become chronically infected. On the other hand, cross-infection between sexual partners and perinatal transmission (although well documented) seem to occur much less frequently than with HBV. Both acute and chronic hepatitis C are clinically mild and usually silent. Indeed, the vast majority (> 95%) of patients with chronic hepatitis C do not recall having had symptomatic hepatitis. The infection is often revealed only many years later when symptoms of chronic liver disease develop, or incidentally through the finding of elevated plasma aminotransferase activities or positive testing for HCV on routine health screening or during investigation of some other condition.

In both the acute and chronic phases, plasma aminotransferases are typically only moderately elevated (often < 500 IU/L, seldom > 1000 IU/L) and characteristically fluctuate (often becoming normal) with a periodicity that ranges from a few weeks to several months or even years. The cause of this fluctuation is unknown but it may reflect an interaction between the host immune response and a cyclical pattern in the life of the virus. Other biochemical parameters are usually normal or only slightly abnormal. Mild to moderate hypergammaglobulinaemia is a frequent finding and autoantibodies can be found at moderate titres in up to 40% of cases, which can present a problem for the differential diagnosis from autoimmune hepatitis (Chapter 6).

Chronic hepatitis C varies widely in severity, from mild non-specific changes in the liver to florid hepatitis with cirrhosis. Plasma biochemical liver tests do not reliably reflect severity, which can usually be assessed only by liver biopsy. Concomitant infection with HCV in other liver disorders such as hepatitis B, schistosomiasis, alcoholic liver disease (Chapter 5) or autoimmune hepatitis (Chapter 6), exacerbates these conditions and there is increasing evidence that HCV may have oncogenic potential (Chapter 7).

HCV SEROLOGY
Infection with HCV is associated with the development of virus-specific

antibodies within a few weeks of exposure to the virus and these persist during the viraemic phase. In acute, self-limited HCV infections, the anti-HCV antibodies disappear shortly after the virus has been cleared. In the majority of HCV-infected individuals, therefore, the presence of anti-HCV antibodies indicates ongoing infection. 'Anti-HCV' comprises a range of antibodies with specificities for different proteins encoded by the viral genome. The specificities of these antibodies vary between infected individuals and at different times during the course of infection. The first commercial anti-HCV enzyme immunoassay (EIA) to be developed was based on detection of antibodies reacting with a recombinant protein synthesised from a sequence corresponding to part of the NS4/NS5 region of the genome (Figure 3.7). It proved to be unreliable, giving false negative results (because it did not detect antibodies reacting with other viral components) as well as frequent false positive results (for other technical reasons). Subsequent technical improvements and development of EIAs that detect antibodies reacting with several different viral components (mainly corresponding to the core, envelope, NS3 and NS5 regions) have provided much more reliable assays. Nevertheless, it is customary to confirm positive anti-HCV tests by supplementary techniques including recombinant immunoblot assays (RIBAs) and detection of viral RNA. The latter requires the use of polymerase chain reaction (PCR) techniques because the viraemia in HCV infection is typically low-grade. Tests for anti-HCV and HCV-RNA are now performed by many routine virology laboratories. Other investigations requiring more rigorous and time-consuming techniques are under-taken mainly in specialised centres. For example, occasionally patients with chronic hepatitis C are anti-HCV positive but negative for HCV-RNA in plasma. However, the virus infects both the liver and peripheral blood mononuclear cells (PBMCs) and, in such individuals, the infection can be confirmed by PCR for HCV-RNA in PBMCs or liver biopsy specimens, or by in situ hybridisation techniques on liver. Quantitative PCR to measure changes in viral load during anti-viral therapy, and serotyping or genotyping to identify strains of the virus that are associated with a better or worse prognosis, may also be performed.

HEPATITIS D

The hepatitis D (Delta) virus (HDV) is a defective pathogen with an RNA genome and a specific protein (the Delta antigen, HDAg) enclosed within an envelope of HBV surface protein (HBsAg). It is wholly dependent on HBV and is acquired by the same routes, either as a co-infection with the initial HBV inoculum or as a super-infection in an individual who is already infected with HBV. The rate of cross-infection between sexual partners seems to be lower than for HBV on its own and the main route of transmission appears to be via the use of unsterilised needles or other medical or cultural practices involving direct blood-to-blood contact. The distribution varies widely around the world. It is highest in the northern parts of South America, the Mediterranean area, some eastern European countries such as Romania and some of the Pacific islands but is surprisingly low in other areas where HBV is endemic, including India, mainland China and most parts of eastern and central Europe. In these and other areas, HDV infection is largely confined to intravenous drug users. However, large-scale programmes of vaccination against HBV and introduction of disposable needles seems to be reducing the incidence of HDV infection.

HDV infection can be acute or chronic. The sequence of events depends to some extent on whether the virus is acquired as a co-infection or as a super-infection in an individual who is already chronically infected with HBV. Co-infection can lead to a biphasic acute hepatitis with an interval of up to six weeks, in which the first episode is due to HBV and the second to HDV (Figure 3.8). Unless tests for HDV are performed, the second episode may be interpreted as a relapse of the HBV-induced illness. In uncomplicated cases, the second episode is often accompanied by clearance of HBV and therefore also of HDV. Super-infected HBV carriers may experience a self-limiting hepatitis followed by clearance of HDV and sometimes also of HBV. More often, such individuals develop chronic HDV infection, which is associated with more severe liver disease and a more rapid progression to cirrhosis. Occasionally, HDV infections can be particularly severe and lead to acute liver failure (Chapter 1), which carries a high mortality.

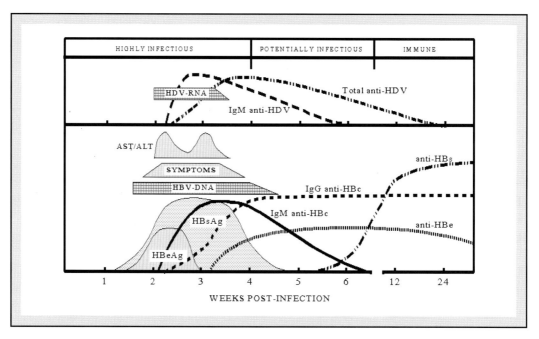

Figure 3.8 Serological events in uncomplicated acute hepatitis D virus (HDV) co-infection with hepatitis B virus

HDV SEROLOGY

RIAs and ELISAs for detection of the HDV antigen (HDAg) and its corresponding IgM and IgG antibodies, and a molecular hybridization method for detection of the viral RNA genome in plasma, have been developed and most of these tests are now commercially available. However, they are performed in only a few specialised laboratories and even these often only test for total anti-HDV antibodies. The serological markers of HDV infection must be measured in conjunction with, and the results interpreted in relation to, the various markers of HBV infection. It is important to note that HDV interferes with HBV replication. In super-infected individuals, this leads to a transient fall in HBsAg titres and often a diminution in titres of other HBV plasma markers accompanied by HBeAg/anti-HBe seroconversion (Figure 3.9). Thus, if testing for anti-HDV is not performed, it is possible to misinterpret HDV super-infection as a spontaneous seroconversion.

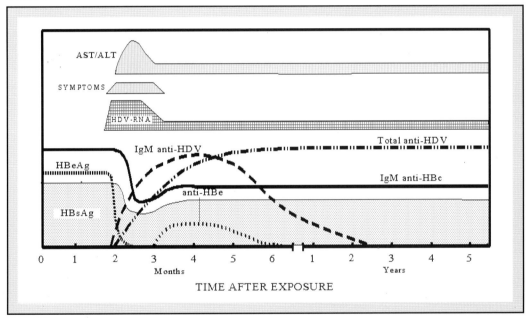

Figure 3.9 Serological events in acute hepatitis D virus (HDV) super-infection in a patient with chronic hepatitis B, with progression to chronic HDV infection.

HEPATITIS E

The hepatitis E virus (HEV) is a positive strand, non-enveloped RNA virus, 27-34 nm in size. Its classification has not yet been fully established but it bears similarities to the caliciviruses and to some togaviruses (such as rubella) and it has been provisionally classified as a new genus, Hepevirus, under the family Calciviridae. It has a world-wide distribution but is particularly noted for large-scale epidemics of hepatitis involving up to tens of thousands of people in developing countries (mainly in tropical and sub-tropical areas). Although there is evidence that HEV can be transmitted parenterally, it is a water-borne virus and infections are predominantly acquired through drinking faeces-contaminated water. Clinically, hepatitis E is very similar to hepatitis A but tends to be more severe and has a greater propensity for development of acute hepatic failure, particularly in pregnant women infected during the third trimester (in whom the mortality is about 20%). Intrauterine HEV infection has been observed, with significant morbidity and mortality in neonates, but in general adults appear to be more susceptible than children.

The incubation period for hepatitis E ranges from 15 to 50 days. There is then usually a prodromal phase of up to ten days associated with generalised symptoms of gastrointestinal upset, followed by the abrupt appearance of jaundice, dark urine and pale stools. Biochemical liver test results are typical of acute viral hepatitis. There is usually a rapid elevation of plasma aminotransferases either immediately preceding, or coinciding with, the appearance of jaundice (Figure 3.10). Viraemia and virus-shedding in stools begins during the incubation and prodromal phases and usually continues for up to ten days during the symptomatic phase. Occasionally the viraemia may be more protracted (up to 100 days) but true chronic infection seems not to occur.

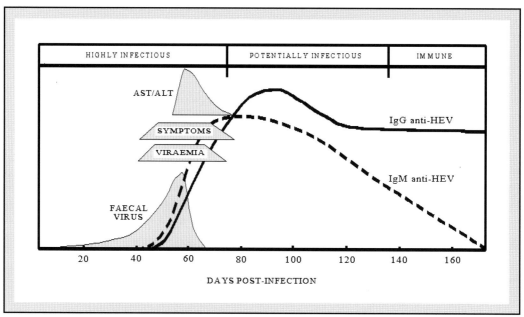

Figure 3.10 Serological events in acute hepatitis E virus (HEV) infection

HEV SEROLOGY

Both IgM and IgG anti-HEV antibodies are detectable early in the course of the disease (Figure 3.10). EIAs for detection of these antibodies are commercially available and are used diagnostically to distinguish between current or recent infection (IgM anti-HEV positive) and previous exposure to the virus (only IgG anti-HEV positive). HEV-RNA can be detected by PCR in blood and stools but this is mainly a research tool and is not used for routine diagnostic purposes.

OTHER VIRUSES

The liver is frequently involved in patients with human immunodeficiency virus (HIV) infection and this is reflected in clinical, radiological imaging, and biochemical abnormalities indicative of liver disease. In almost all cases, however, these findings relate to malignancies or to a wide range of opportunistic or concomitant viral, bacterial, fungal or parasitic infections in the immunocompromised host rather than to HIV per se. Non-Hodgkin's lymphoma of the liver is a relatively frequent tumour in HIV-infected patients. Kaposi's sarcoma may also affect the liver. Co-infection with HBV or HCV is particularly associated with severe liver disease. This is especially true of co-infection with HCV, which results in an unusually rapid progression to cirrhosis and liver failure, higher mortality and increased risk of hepatocellular carcinoma (Chapter 7) compared with chronic hepatitis C without HIV infection.

Other viruses, such as the hepatitis G virus (GB-C/HGV), Epstein-Barr virus (EBV) and cytomegalovirus (CMV), only rarely cause hepatitis, although CMV infection is a particular problem in liver transplant recipients (Chapter 9). The arboviruses and arenaviruses are important in those parts of the world (e.g., continental Africa) where they are endemic, but need also to be considered in patients who develop hepatitis after travelling to such areas. Because of their clinical features, other viral infections that may occasionally involve the liver, such as those caused by coxsackie, echo, rubella, herpes simplex and varicella zoster viruses, do not usually present a major problem in the differential diagnosis of hepatitis but need to be borne in mind.

TREMATODE AND CESTODE INFECTIONS

The trematodes that mainly infect humans are the blood flukes (*Schistosoma sp.*) and the liver flukes (*Clonorchis, Fasciola* and, in certain parts of the Far East, *Opisthorchis sp.*), while by far the most important cestodes capable of invading the liver are the Echinococcus sp. tapeworms. Liver disorders associated with Taenia infections (usually *T. saginata or T. solium*) are relatively rare.

SCHISTOSOMIASIS

Six species of schistosome worms are known to infect humans: *S. mansoni, S. haematobium, S. japonicum, S. intercalatum, S. mekongi and S. mattheei*. All require a fresh-water snail as an intermediate host. Each inhabits a particular species of snail and the geographical distribution of the different schistomes is governed by the range of their molluscan hosts. The two most important species that infect the liver are *S. mansoni and S. japonicum*. The former occurs in most areas where schistosomiasis is endemic while the latter is mainly confined to parts of the Far East. Schistosomiasis is spread through contamination of water in which the snails live by faeces containing the eggs of the parasite. The eggs hatch to produce a motile organism (the miracidium) which infects the snail. The miracidia become sporocytes which reproduce and eventually develop into free-swimming infective cercariae that are shed from the snails during daylight hours and can penetrate the skin or (if ingested) mucous membranes in the gut. During this process the cerceriae become schistosomules that migrate through the blood vessels and eventually reach the liver where they develop to maturity. The hepatic disease is due to a host immune reaction to the parasite. Fibrosis is the dominant histological feature and has a characteristic pattern known as 'pipe-stem' or Symmer's fibrosis. A proportion of patients develop more severe disease with inflammation and necrosis of the hepatic parenchyma but it appears that in the majority of such cases this is due to concomitant infection with the hepatitis B or C viruses.

The laboratory findings are very variable and depend on the stage of the disease (which may remain asymptomatic for many years) and its severity. They range from only mild elevations in plasma ALP and GGT to abnormalities in all of the biochemical liver tests, including elevated aminotransferases and bilirubin concentrations. Plasma IgG is often increased, as well as IgM to a lesser extent, but IgA is usually normal. A variety of organ-specific and non-organ-specific autoantibodies (Chapter 6) have been reported in patients with schistosomiasis. These are of uncertain diagnostic significance but there is evidence that liver-specific autoimmune reactions may play a role in the hepatic parenchymal damage.

Diagnosis requires the microscopic demonstration of ova in stools, or in liver or rectal biopsies. Ultrasonography is being increasingly used to diagnose Symmer's fibrosis. A skin test may be used for screening purposes but is prone to giving false-positive results. A wide range of serological tests is available but none is sufficiently reliable to replace direct demonstration of the parasite.

LIVER FLUKES

These organisms colonise the biliary tract and the laboratory findings are those normally associated with large bile duct obstruction. The extent of the plasma biochemical abnormalities depends on the stage and severity of the infection (which is often asymptomatic). Anaemia is a common finding and a marked eosinophilia may be observed, especially in the early stages of Clonorchis infection. The latter predisposes to cholangiocarcinoma (Chapter 7) and is often associated with pancreatitis, which may complicate interpretation of the laboratory findings. Skin tests and various serological tests for liver fluke infestations are available but, so far, none has proved sufficiently reliable to replace direct demonstration of parasite ova in stool specimens for definitive diagnosis.

HYDATID DISEASE

In cestode infections, the tapeworms become trapped in the liver (almost always in the centrilobular veins of the right lobe) where they develop into fully encapsulated hydatid cysts. Their manifestation is usually clinical, the biochemical liver tests often being normal. However, hydatid cysts grow at a rate of about 1 cm per year and eventually compress the surrounding liver tissue. Depending on the precise location of the cyst, this can lead to mechanical obstruction of the intrahepatic blood and bile flow, resulting in congestion and cholestasis with biochemical liver test abnormalities suggestive of biliary obstruction. Occasionally there may be a superimposed secondary infection or a cyst may rupture, leading to cholangitis and a reactive hepatitis with elevated aminotransferases. Diagnosis depends on serology. There are many tests available, but each is subject to wide intra- and inter-laboratory variations and the current recommendation is that a combination of two or more tests should be employed.

GRANULOMATOUS LIVER DISEASES

In Europe and North America, the commonest causes of granulomatous liver disease are sarcoidosis and tuberculosis. The latter, together with various other bacterial, as well as fungal and parasitic, infections are important in the tropics. However, granulomas in the liver are also seen with variable frequency in association with a very wide range of other conditions (Figure 3.11) and are a characteristic of primary biliary cirrhosis (PBC, Chapter 6). With few exceptions (notably PBC), the biochemical liver test abnormalities are fairly unremarkable and are generally not very helpful. Diagnoses are usually based on liver biopsy findings in conjunction with identification of the primary disorder. The most frequent biochemical abnormality is an elevated ALP. Marked hyperbilirubinaemia is rare and plasma aminotransferase activities are usually normal or only slightly increased.

Granulomatous liver disease		
Idiopathic disorders	**Infections**	**Drugs**
Crohn's disease	Bacterial	Aspirin
Erythema nodosum	*Brucellosis*	Chlorpropamide
Hodgkin's disease	*Leprosy*	Diazepam
Polymyalgia rheumatica	*Listeriosis*	Hydralazine
Primary biliary cirrhosis	Fungal	Methyldopa
Sarcoidosis	*Coccidioidomycosis*	Penicillins
Ulcerative colitis	*Histoplasmosis*	Phenytoin
	Parasitic	Phenylbutazone
	Schistosomiasis	Procainamide
	Toxocariasis	Quinidine
	Rickettsial	Sulphonamides
	Spirochaetal	Thiazides
	Viral	Tolbutamide
	Cytomegalovirus	
	Epstein-Barr virus	

Figure 3.11 Some causes of granulomatous liver disease

Sarcoidosis is a multisystem granulomatous disease of unknown cause. More than 90% of patients have pulmonary manifestations. Liver involvement occurs in 10-20% of cases but jaundice is uncommon and marked elevations of the plasma aminotransferases are rare. Hyperglobulinaemia, due mainly to elevated plasma IgG, is a frequent finding along with low titres of a variety of autoantibodies (e.g., anti-nuclear and anti-smooth muscle) and high titres of antibodies against a wide range of common pathogens (e.g., rubella, coliform bacteria), reflecting a generalised heightened immunoresponsiveness. Diagnosis is based on a spectrum of clinicopathological findings in various tissues including the lungs and mediastinal lymph nodes. The Kveim-Siltzbach skin test, involving intradermal injection of an extract of spleen tissue from a patient with active sarcoidosis, was used diagnostically but is now only of historical interest owing to its propensity to give false-negative results and limited availability of the antigen. Plasma angiotensin-converting enzyme (ACE) activities are elevated in cases of active sarcoidosis and are a useful marker of disease activity but are of little value in diagnosing hepatic sarcoidosis because increased are found in several other liver disorders.

Hepatic granulomas are almost always found in acute miliary tuberculosis but biochemical and haematological changes are non-specific. In other forms of tuberculosis, the incidence of liver involvement varies but is usually not greater than 20% and is often not clinically obvious. Diagnosis depends on a positive Mantoux skin test, but a negative result does not exclude tuberculosis.

LEPTOSPIROSIS

Leptospirosis was relatively rare in Western Europe and North America but has recently been on the increase, and sporadic outbreaks are not uncommon elsewhere in the world. It is caused by *Leptospira interrogans* organisms which are carried by rats and other feral mammals but domestic animals may also be hosts. Transmission is normally via animal bites or contact with their urine or faeces. The illness usually follows a biphasic course and ranges from a mild febrile condition to a severe (often fatal) form with profound jaundice. The jaundice is not secondary to hepatocellular necrosis, which is minimal. Rather, it appears to be related to impairment of bilirubin transport. This severe form (Weil's disease) is usually caused by *L. icterohaemorrhagiae* but may also be due to *L. canis* (carried by dogs) or other species.

The most striking biochemical finding in Weil's disease is a marked conjugated hyperbilirubinaemia with bilirubinuria. The plasma ALP and aminotransferase activities are usually elevated only to a mild to moderate extent but either or both may be markedly raised and the condition may therefore be confused with either biliary obstruction or acute viral hepatitis. There is usually a degree of renal impairment and urinalysis reveals proteinuria, casts and increased numbers of erythrocytes and leucocytes. Uraemia may develop, with urea concentrations rising to 20-40 mmol/L. The main haematological finding is a leucocytosis. Anaemia due to intravascular haemolysis frequently develops in the later stages and may be severe. Prothrombin times and platelet counts are usually normal. Diagnosis depends mainly on demonstrating anti-leptospiral antibodies in plasma, for the organism itself appears in the blood only during the early stages of infection. Specific tests are available for these antibodies, which usually appear during the second week of the illness and increase rapidly in titre over the following three weeks. Thereafter, titres decline but the patient may remain seropositive for several years.

OTHER INFECTIOUS DISEASES OF THE LIVER

LIVER ABSCESSES

Hepatic abscesses are broadly classified according to whether they are caused by bacterial (pyogenic abscesses) or amoebic infections. They tend to occur much more frequently in older adults (often with pre-existing biliary disease) than in the young. Pyogenic abscesses may be caused by infections with either aerobic or anaerobic organisms. Identification of the responsible organism by blood culture can be difficult, partly because multiple infections are not uncommon. Amoebic infections of the liver are much more common in tropical countries than in temperate zones. Diagnosis is usually made by ultrasonography or other imaging techniques and relies on serology, i.e., the demonstration of IgM and IgG antibodies against the organism. Negative serology excludes amoebiasis but a positive test is not necessarily diagnostic of current infection.

Whatever the cause of the abscess, the most frequently found biochemical abnormality is a high ALP activity. Plasma bilirubin concentrations are usually only moderately raised (less markedly and less often in patients with amoebic abscesses than in those with pyogenic abscesses). Plasma aminotransferase activities tend to be near normal but may be elevated 3- to 4-fold and, in that event, are considered a poor prognostic sign. Hypoalbuminaemia and hypergammaglobulinaemia are frequent findings. The haematological picture includes a marked leucocytosis, raised ESR, anaemia and (in protracted illnesses) prolongation of INR. The most important differential diagnosis of hepatic abscess is from hepatocellular carcinoma (HCC) and it is therefore worthwhile to measure the α-fetoprotein (AFP), although a normal AFP does not necessarily exclude HCC (Chapter 7). Among other laboratory tests that might be performed, perhaps the most useful is the vitamin B12. High concentrations of vitamin B12 (often exceeding 1000 ng/L) are very common in patients with hepatic abscesses, although they are not specific for this condition because similar concentrations can also be seen in patients with malignant liver disease and in some other disorders.

FUNGAL INFECTIONS
Disseminated fungal infections that involve the liver are seen fairly frequently in tropical areas, but (with a few exceptions) in other countries hepatic involvement is mainly confined to immunocompromised individuals receiving chemotherapy for malignancies or immunosuppressive therapy related to organ grafting or autoimmune diseases and in patients with AIDS. In many cases the diagnoses can be made by serological or skin tests but, in others, histological demonstration of the infection is required and is often revealed only at autopsy. Several, such as blastomycosis, coccidioidomycosis and histoplasmosis, are important causes of granulomatous diseases (Figure 3.10) and may be confused with hepatic tuberculosis or sarcoidosis. The biochemical liver tests are usually only mildly abnormal, but may occasionally be severely deranged. Aspergillosis has been associated with thrombosis of the hepatic venous system (Budd-Chiari syndrome), with markedly elevated bilirubin, ALP and aminotransferases, while similar derangements can be seen in disseminated cryptococcosis which has been misdiagnosed as primary sclerosing cholangitis (Chapter 6). Hepatic candidiasis is common in immuno-

compromised hosts and is a major problem, especially in liver graft recipients. It should be suspected in any immuno-compromised individual with unexplained pyrexia, especially if the ALP activity is markedly elevated, but it is important to note that only about half of those infected will have positive blood cultures. In the remainder, diagnosis requires a liver biopsy.

SYSTEMIC BACTERIAL INFECTIONS
Systemic bacterial infections can cause hepatic dysfunction even when the liver is not directly involved. Their importance in the present context relates to the likelihood that the hepatic abnormalities may distract attention from serious extrahepatic disease. In neonates and young children, a sudden and profound conjugated hyperbilirubinaemia can be the first evidence of systemic infection, e.g., secondary to an *E. coli* urinary tract infection. Usually this is the main (often the only) biochemical liver abnormality. In adults, a wide range of Gram-positive and Gram-negative bacteria can cause jaundice. Such patients are usually very ill and the hyperbilirubinaemia will often be accompanied by a leucocytosis, normochromic anaemia and a raised ESR. Hypoalbuminaemia and hypergamma-globulinaemia are common. Plasma ALP activity may be raised (occasionally markedly) in the absence of jaundice and may be the only abnormality detected. Plasma aminotransferase activities are generally normal or only slightly elevated in these situations.

FURTHER READING

Eyster ME. Effect of HIV infection on hepatitis C. Viral Hepatitis Rev 1998; **4:** 189-206.

Jordan P, Webbe G, Sturrock RF. Human Schistosomiasis. Wallingford: CAB International, 1993: 465 pp.

Reesink HW. Hepatitis C virus. 2nd ed. Karger, London; 1998: 270 pp.

Webbe G. Recent developments in cestode research. Trans Roy Soc Trop Med Hyg 1995; **89:** 345-6.

Zuckerman AJ, Thomas HC, eds. Viral hepatitis. Churchill Livingstone, London: 1993: 590 pp.

Chapter 4.

Metabolic Liver Disorders

INTRODUCTION

A wide range of inherited metabolic disorders affects the liver either directly or indirectly. Although the individual conditions are relatively rare, collectively they comprise a significant proportion of liver disease, particularly in children. They range from diseases associated with excessive tissue storage of iron (haemochromatosis) or copper (Wilson disease), through abnormalities of carbohydrate, lipid and bilirubin metabolism, to the mitochondrial and peroxisomal disorders. It is essential to diagnose these disorders rapidly, particularly in neonates, because many are treatable and can have severe long-term sequelae if appropriate management is not initiated promptly. Although definitive diagnosis usually requires specialist expertise, including the use of molecular or cellular techniques in some of the conditions, most of the disorders are associated with characteristic findings on simple laboratory testing that should raise the level of suspicion when a patient with clinical evidence of liver disease is seen.

IRON OVERLOAD SYNDROMES

Iron overload can be considered to exist when total body iron stores exceed 1 mmol/kg body weight and may be caused by excessive iron absorption from the gut or from parenteral iron loading by repeated blood transfusion. Iron accumulates initially in the parenchymal cells of the liver and in the cells of the reticuloendothelial system, but excessive iron deposits may also be found in the heart, pancreas and other organs in the later stages of the disease. The generic term haemochromatosis encompasses all the iron overload syndromes and these can be sub-divided into primary, hereditary haemochromatosis, and secondary, which includes a variety of disorders (Figure 4.1).

HEREDITARY HAEMOCHROMATOSIS

Hereditary haemochromatosis (HH) is probably the commonest cause of non-iatrogenic iron overload. It is inherited as an autosomal recessive disorder with an overall prevalence ranging from 1 in 200 to 1 in 400 in Caucasian populations. A prevalence of 1 in 300 would imply nearly 10% of the population being carriers. Although the disease was first described over 100 years ago the structural and functional nature of the defect has not yet been defined. HH was initially identified because of the association of marked liver iron loading with diabetes mellitus which is the commonest presenting feature. In the pre-insulin era, the prognosis of patients with HH was poor. The introduction first of insulin and second of venesection therapy has significantly improved the mortality and morbidity of the condition. Although HH is an autosomal recessive disorder clinical presentation is more common in males and older females. This is likely to be due to a greater iron loading in males and the effects of menstrual blood loss in younger females. Weakness, arthritis and liver disease (cirrhosis) are the commonest presenting features whilst men with HH may also present with hypogonadotrophic hypogo-nadism (testicular atrophy, gynaecomastia and loss of libido) and cardiomyopathy (usually in the later stages). The successful treatment of the acute complications of haemochromatosis has revealed an incidence of hepatocellular carcinoma in HH many times that of the normal population and this now accounts for a significant proportion of the mortality associated with HH when cirrhosis has supervened. A juvenile form of HH, which is more rapidly progressive, has been described with major iron deposits in the heart and endocrine glands, particularly the pituitary.

Iron overload syndromes
Increased iron absorption
Hereditary haemochromatosis
Alcohol related cirrhosis   Porphyria cutanea tarda
Massive ineffective erythropoiesis (e.g., sideroblastic anaemia)
Bantu siderosis
Iatrogenic due to inappropriate or excessive therapy
Parenteral iron overload
Ineffective erythropoiesis (e.g., thalassaemia major)
Hypoplastic erythropoiesis (e.g., chronic renal failure, aplastic and myelodysplastic anaemias)

Figure 4.1 Iron overload syndromes

The gene responsible for HH is called HFE and was identified by positional cloning on the short arm of chromosome 6 after initial reports of linkage with the HLA class 1 genes. HFE shows strong homology to classical and non-classical class I genes and has been shown to form a physical association with the transferrin receptor. A mutation (CYS 282TYR) has been identified in the HFE gene in over 90% of patients with HH in the UK, but in lower proportions (60-70%) of patients in southern European countries such as Italy. A second mutation (HIS63ASP) has been identified, but this mutation is present in up to 20% of control populations and when homozygous rarely causes significant iron overload. Approximately 3% of patients with clinically significant HH carry one copy each of CYS 282TYR and HIS63ASP and are known as compound heterozygotes. These patients have only a minimal increase in iron stores but may still be symptomatic with tiredness and minor changes in liver biochemistry (see below) The manner in which the gene product leads to the increased iron absorption from a normal diet is not known, but it has been suggested that the mutant protein fails to bind the transferrin receptor and this leads to faulty sensing of body iron stores by intestinal absorbing cells. Overall, the phenotype is very variable and there is a 10-fold variation in body iron stores.

The classic liver biochemistry tests are of little value in the diagnosis of HH. The results are often only mildly abnormal and give no real indication of the nature of the underlying disorder. Up to one quarter of patients with HH have a plasma iron concentration within the reference range (10-30 μmol/L) and conversely, it is not uncommon for healthy individuals to have plasma iron concentrations in excess of 30 μmol/L. Transferrin saturation is almost always above the reference range (20-50%) and a saturation of greater than 75% is probably required before significant iron accumulation in hepatocytes occurs. However, the false positive rate on the basis of this cut-off can be up to 30% as increased transferrin saturation can also occur in liver disease, following oral or parenteral iron supplementation and in some erythrocyte disorders. Plasma ferritin is typically greater than 1000 μg/L in symptomatic patients but may be only slightly elevated (300-500 μg/L) in asymptomatic subjects. Other causes of a raised plasma ferritin, such as inflammation need to be excluded. Figure 4.2 contrasts the findings for plasma tests of iron metabolism in HH and secondary iron overload.

If the initial tests indicate markedly increased iron stores then a liver biopsy should be used to confirm the diagnosis. Appropriate staining of the sections will reveal the excessive deposition of iron in hepatocytes and Kupffer cells, but a quantitative measurement of the liver iron content should also be made. Normal liver usually contains less than 25 μmol iron/g dry weight, whereas in HH the hepatic iron concentration is generally in excess of 200 μmol/g. There is a tendency for the liver iron concentration to increase with age and the hepatic iron index, calculated by dividing the hepatic iron concentration in micromoles by the patient's age in years, was introduced to attempt to compensate for this. A hepatic iron index > 2 is characteristic of HH.

Laboratory findings in iron overload		
Test (reference range)	Hereditary haemochromatosis	Secondary iron overload
Standard LFTs	Mildly abnormal	Variable
Plasma iron (10-30 µmol/L)	Usually > 30	Usually > 30
TIBC (45-70 µmol/L)	Usually normal	Normal, very occasionally >70
Transferrin saturation (20 - 50%)	>50% often >70%	Usually normal, occasionally > 60%
Plasma ferritin (< 200 µg/L)	>1000	Usually < 500, often normal

Figure 4.2 Typical laboratory findings in hereditary haemochromatosis and secondary iron overload

Using a restriction enzyme which cuts the wild type of the HFE gene at CYS but not at TYR in the most frequent mutated form, a relatively simple molecular assay has now been developed that can identify patients with the CYS282TYR mutation. (Figure 4.3) The benefits of such an assay is the detection of heterozygotes and asymptomatic homozygotes in patient's families. Screening of high risk populations, such as patients with diabetes, has been proposed using a combination of plasma ferritin and transferrin saturation, backed up by molecular assays. Initial studies, however, have reported a low detection rate for HH and the value of screening apart from in families with known cases of HH has been questioned.

The primary treatment for HH is venesection which should be performed weekly, by removing 500-600 mL of blood on each occasion. The aim of treatment is to bring the plasma ferritin concentration within the reference range (< 200 µg/L) and the plasma iron to < 30 µmol/L. The plasma iron begins to fall only when available iron stores are depleted which may take 1-2 years of therapy in patients with markedly increased iron stores.

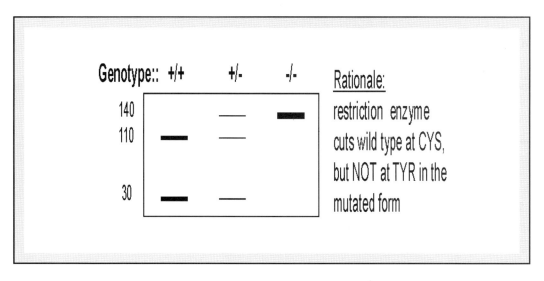

Figure 4.3 Detection of the CYS282TYR mutation in hereditary haemochromatosis
The restriction enzyme cuts the wild type at CYS, but not at TYR in the mutated form

SECONDARY IRON OVERLOAD

A proportion of patients with cirrhosis (due to causes other than HH) will show some increased iron deposition in the liver. This may be accompanied by raised plasma ferritin and occasionally transferrin saturation, but these changes are seldom of the magnitude seen in HH (Figure 4.2). Although such abnormalities may be found in cirrhosis of any cause, they are most common in alcohol-related liver disease and particularly in males with porphyria cutanea tarda (PCT). It has been shown that the incidence of HH is no higher in patients with alcohol-related liver disease than in the normal population. The mechanism behind the apparent excess iron absorption in these patients is unclear but may be related to pancreatic exocrine insufficiency or to a direct promoting effect of alcohol on iron absorption. In general, dietary iron overload is rare, with the notable exception of the Bantu of southern Africa, who develop a syndrome similar to HH that is related to the consumption of alcoholic beverages brewed in iron pots in people with a genetic susceptibility to absorb excess dietary iron.

Other conditions in which secondary iron overload is a feature include the haemolytic anaemias (particularly those due to ineffective erythropoiesis) associated with thalassaemia major, congenital spherocytosis and the hereditary sideroblastic and sickle-cell anaemias. Secondary iron overload is also common in patients receiving multiple blood transfusions, e.g., chronic renal dialysis patients, but in contrast to the iron loading related to ineffective erythropoiesis (which is predominantly parenchymal) parenterally acquired iron tends to accumulate in reticuloendothelial cells where it does not adversely affect the liver until the iron burden is so great that it spills over into the parenchymal cells.

COPPER STORAGE DISEASE

Abnormal accumulation of copper in the liver and other tissues occurs in one well-documented genetic disorder (Wilson disease) and in a number of acquired conditions, including Indian childhood cirrhosis.

WILSON DISEASE

Wilson disease is an inborn error of metabolism that results in abnormal deposition of copper, first in the liver and then progressively in the kidneys, brain, eyes and other tissues. It is inherited as an autosomal recessive disorder with an approximate worldwide prevalence of 1:200,000 for homozygotes and 1:200 for heterozygotes. Accumulation of copper in the eyes is associated with the appearance of Kayser-Fleischer rings in the cornea (detectable by slit-lamp examination); accumulation in the brain leads to the development of neurological symptoms and a characteristic neuropathy. The onset of symptoms may occur at any time, but the peak of onset is in adolescence and cases in children less than three years old or in adults over 50 years are rare. The hepatic manifestations vary widely at presentation, from the silent development of cirrhosis to a more acute onset of hepatitis often accompanied by haemolysis and evidence of renal tubular dysfunction and which may rapidly progress to fulminant hepatic failure. Accurate diagnosis is essential as early institution of treatment with copper chelators (D-penicillamine being the agent of choice) is usually very effective for arresting, preventing the progression to cirrhosis or neurological symptoms and reversing much of the neurological damage already present at diagnosis.

The defect in Wilson disease has now been attributed to a gene designated ATP7B on chromosome 13 (located at 13q14.3) with a resulting failure in ATP-ase dependent copper excretion. Several common defects have been identified which account for up to 50% of cases of Wilson's disease, but new mutations continue to be identified and over 60 are known to date. Most patients are compound heterozygotes, carrying a different mutation on each chromosome 13

Whilst the presence of Kayser-Fleischer rings in the cornea should raise a strong clinical suspicion of Wilson disease, these are not invariably present, particularly in children presenting in early infancy. Diagnosis therefore requires assessment of copper status (Figure 4.4). The main non-invasive tests for copper metabolism are measurement of plasma and urinary copper and plasma caeruloplasmin, a blue copper-containing glycoprotein synthesized in the liver. About 90% of Wilson disease patients have plasma caeruloplasmin concentrations < 200 mg/L (reference range 200-400 mg/L) and the rest have concentrations < 300 mg/L, i.e., in the lower half of the reference range. The total plasma copper concentration is below the reference range in a significant proportion of patients but the overlap with other diseases reduces the diagnostic significance of the results. Some 90% (10-25 μmol/L) of the copper in normal plasma is bound irreversibly to caeruloplasmin, the remainder (< 2 μmol/L) being loosely bound to albumin or to amino acids. This latter fraction is termed the 'free' copper and may be elevated 10-fold or more in Wilson disease. A 'free' plasma copper concentration greater than 7 μmol/L is virtually diagnostic of Wilson disease but this is only found in approximately 50% of patients. Urinary copper excretion in normal subjects is low (0.5-2.0 μmol/24h) and patients with Wilson disease may have a basal copper excretion up to 10-fold higher than this (up to 20 μmol/24h).

Laboratory findings in Wilson disease			
	Symptomatic		Asymptomatic
	Insidious onset	Acute onset	
Standard liver biochemistry tests	Abnormal but variable	Severely deranged	Usually normal
Plasma copper			
Total (10 - 30 μmol/L)	Variable	> 30	Variable
Free (< 2 μmol/L)	>10	> 10	> 2
Plasma caeruloplasmin (160 - 350 mg/L)	< 200	< 200	< 300
Urinary copper (0.25 - 0.75 μmol/24h)	> 2	> 15	> 1
Hepatic copper (< 1 μmol/g dry weight)	> 4	> 4	1 - 4
D-penicillamine challenge test	> 20 fold increase in urine copper	Not known	> 10 fold increase in urine copper

Figure 4.4 **Typical laboratory findings in Wilson disease (normal ranges in parentheses)**

There are difficulties, however, in interpreting the results of the non-invasive tests of copper status in patients presenting acutely with evidence of severe hepatocellular necrosis or fulminant hepatic failure. Because caeruloplasmin is synthesized by the liver, any condition in which overall hepatic function is impaired may lead to a decreased plasma caeruloplasmin concentration. Also, because the normal pathway of copper excretion is in the bile, severe hepatic necrosis in the presence of chronic cholestasis will cause release of stored copper from the liver and high plasma and urinary copper concentrations may be seen. Urinary copper excretion is often increased in patients with fulminant hepatic failure due to other causes, but seldom exceeds 15 μmol/24h, whilst in fulminant Wilson disease, urinary copper excretion can exceed 30 μmol/24h.

The two tests with the greatest discriminatory power for the diagnosis of Wilson disease are the measurement of urinary copper excretion following administration of D-penicillamine and assay of hepatic copper content. The D-penicillamine challenge test involves collection of two 24 hour urine samples for copper estimation before and after administration of 0.5g of D-penicillamine. In normal subjects or patients with liver disease other than Wilson disease the post-penicillamine copper excretion seldom exceeds 20 μmol/24h whilst in virtually all Wilson patients the copper excretion is higher than this. In children the penicillamine challenge test has been found to be the most discriminating test in the diagnosis of Wilson disease. The normal copper concentration in the liver is less than 1 μmol/g dry weight of tissue. In untreated patients with Wilson disease, hepatic copper content is almost always greater than 1 μmol/g and can be as high as 40 μmol/g. However, the copper is not deposited uniformly throughout the liver so that some samples may have only mildly raised concentrations. Hepatic copper content can also be elevated in other, mainly cholestatic, liver diseases and a mildly raised value cannot be considered to be diagnostic unless associated with a very low plasma caeruloplasmin concentration. Other tests such as the clearance rate of radioactively labelled copper are now seldom used.

In family studies, detection of heterozygotes for Wilson disease has been difficult. The identification of the gene and development of molecular assays based on single strand conformation polymorphism (SSCP) on sequencing permits the screening of most families, although in some patients with classic Wilson disease no mutations in the ATP7B gene have been found. Because early institution of D-penicillamine therapy is effective for arresting the progress of the disease all first degree relatives of patients with Wilson disease should be screened to detect siblings with asymptomatic disease.

Some 20% of patients receiving D-penicillamine can develop sensitivity reactions to the drug at any stage, but particularly in the early stages of therapy. Standard liver biochemistry tests and full blood count should be measured at 2-4 week intervals for the first six months as leucopenia and thrombocytopenia can develop. Urine should be regularly tested for protein as D-penicillamine can cause a form of nephrotic syndrome or Goodpasture's syndrome.

SECONDARY COPPER OVERLOAD
In most individuals excessive oral intake of copper rarely leads to serious hepatotoxicity. In India and parts of South-East Asia many cases of cirrhosis have been found in whom the hepatic copper content was elevated to levels intermediate between those found in asymptomatic and symptomatic Wilson disease. However, the histological appearance of the liver is unlike that seen in Wilson disease and the condition was labelled Indian childhood cirrhosis. The high copper content of the liver appears to come from prolonged high copper intake either from natural sources or from milk stored in copper vessels. As not all children exposed to the copper sources develop cirrhosis, an underlying genetic susceptibility has been proposed. Indian childhood cirrhosis is a severe and often fatal condition affecting children under ten years of age with a peak onset at between one and three years. Early treatment with D-penicillamine has been shown to reduce mortality and partially reverse the liver damage. Over recent years nearly 20 cases with similar pathological features with or without identifiable environmental sources of excess copper have been reported in Europe, Australia and the USA, in families with no known Asian ancestors. It has been proposed that these disorders would be better named 'copper associated liver disease in childhood'.

Standard biochemical liver tests show marked abnormalities indicating hepatocellular necrosis with a variable degree of cholestasis. The plasma immunoglobulins are usually elevated and smooth-muscle antibodies are positive in up to half of the patients. The condition can be confused at presentation with either acute viral hepatitis or autoimmune hepatitis. Assessment of copper status may reveal elevations in plasma and urinary copper, but rarely to the same extent as in Wilson disease. Plasma caeruloplasmin is usually normal except in the fulminant phase when hepatic synthetic function is reduced. Definitive diagnosis is made histologically on positive orcein staining for copper-associated protein in the presence of micronodular cirrhosis and intracytoplasmic Mallory bodies.

A1-ANTITRYPSIN DEFICIENCY

α1-Antitrypsin (α1-AT) is a glycoprotein synthesised by the liver and is a member of the serpin (serine proteinase inhibitor) family of proteins. Originally it was thought that its major function was the inhibition of trypsin (hence the name), but it is now known that the preferred substrate is elastase and in many texts the term 'α1-protease inhibitor' is used. Deficiency of α1-AT was originally identified in association with early onset emphysema and a link between α1-AT deficiency and liver disease was found subsequently. Liver disease associated with α1-AT deficiency accounts for up to 10% of patients presenting to paediatric hepatologists. There are significant variations in the prevalence of α1-AT deficiency amongst ethnic groups, Caucasians having the highest prevalence (approximately 1 in 2000) and African and Middle Eastern peoples the lowest. Approximately 10-20% of cases of α1-AT deficiency present with features of liver disease in infancy, but asymptomatic elevations of plasma aminotransferases occur in up to 75% of affected individuals in the first year of life. The clinical presentation in patients presenting before six months of age resembles neonatal hepatitis, whereas in older individuals cirrhosis may be the predominant feature. There is a higher incidence of hepatocellular carcinoma in α1-AT deficient subjects than in the normal population, particularly in men over 50 years of age.

Human α1-AT comprises a single chain of 394 amino acids with carbohydrate side chains and has a molecular weight of 52kDa. The gene encoding α1-AT is located on chromosome 14 (14q32.1) and over 90 genetically determined variants of α1-AT have now been reported. The majority of these are exceedingly rare and are associated with normal amounts of functional enzyme. The conventional nomenclature defines individual phenotype by the letters Pi followed by an alphabetical code relating to the mobility of the variant on isoelectric focusing gels. The commonest normal variant found in all populations is designated M (medium) and can be further sub-divided into at least eight subtypes (M1, M2, M3, etc.). There are a number of mutations that result in varying degrees of α1-AT deficiency, the two commonest being designated S (slow) and Z (ultraslow). Rarer mutations are identified by the place name locating the birthplace of the oldest individual tested in a family (e.g., MPittsburgh). Figure. 4.5 details the predominant mutations found in Caucasian populations and the disease susceptibility. Where a mutation results in a frame-shift no immunoreactive protein is formed and these are referred to as null variants.

Liver disease is predominantly associated with the PiZZ phenotype, although several rare variants have also been reported in which liver damage occurs i.e. MDalton, SIiyama. The Z mutation results in hepatocytes secreting only 10-15% of the normal amount of α1-AT. Aggregates of α1-AT can be demonstrated in the endoplasmic reticulum of hepatocytes as diastase-resistant PAS (periodic acid-Schiff) positive granules. The aggregation occurs because the Z mutation is located at the base of the reactive loop of the enzyme resulting in dimerization and subsequent polymerization of the molecule. Additionally the Z variant has reduced capacity for binding elastase and therefore the liver damage may be a combination of α1-AT deposition and unopposed elastase activity. There is still, however, considerable debate about the exact mechanism of liver disease in α1-AT deficiency. The wide variation in disease severity and the concordance in severity in siblings affected may indicate the co-existence of a second genetic factor predisposing to liver damage.

α-1 antitrypsin deficiency		
Allele	**Mutation**	**Disease susceptibility**
M	Wild type	None
M_1	Ala^{213}GCG to ValGTG	None
M_2	Arg^{101}CGT to HisCAT	None
F	Arg^{223}CGT to CysTGT	None
S	Glu^{264}AAA to ValGTA	Lung disease
Z	Glu^{342}GAG to LysAAG	Lung and liver disease
M$_{malton}$	Phe^{52}TTC to delete TTC	Liver disease
Null	Various deletions etc.	Lung disease
Phenotype	**Approximate frequency (%)**	**Plasma α1-AT concentration (% of normal)**
MM	90	100
MS	5	60
MZ	3	60
SS	1	60
SZ	0.2	40
ZZ	0.05	15

Figure 4.5 Common mutations in the α1-AT gene and the clinical consequences of resulting phenotypes

α1-AT constitutes approximately 90% of the α1-globulin band on serum protein electrophoresis and its deficiency can therefore be revealed by the marked reduction in this band. Estimation of α1-AT by immunochemical techniques can identify a quantitative deficiency of α1-AT in plasma. Since α1-AT is an acute phase reactant, the plasma concentration may be artefactually increased into the reference range in response to inflammatory stimuli or in liver disease itself. On the other hand, artefactually low concentrations may occur in acute hepatic necrosis or protein-losing enteropathies. Determination of the phenotype by isoelectric focusing (IEF) on acrylamide gels is, therefore, the best approach to confirming or excluding the diagnosis in patients with liver disease. The reduced concentration of protein associated with the Z mutation can make it difficult to see the Z band in PiZZ individuals but determining the phenotype of the parents will usually confirm the PiZZ phenotype in the affected patients (Figure 4.6)

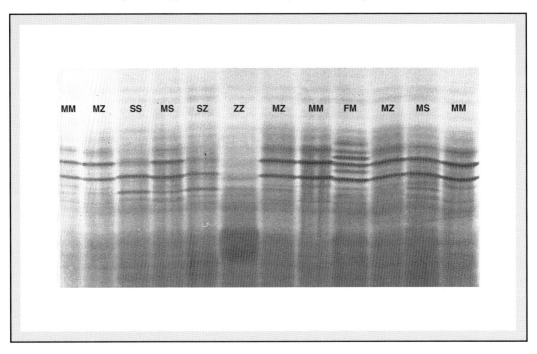

Figure 4.6 Isoelectric focusing for determination of α1-AT phenotypes

Knowledge of the specific gene mutations associated with the S and Z mutations has permitted the development of molecular assays using either the restriction fragment length polymorphism (RFLP) or amplification refractory mutation system (ARMS) techniques. These techniques can be used to provide a prenatal diagnosis from chorionic villus samples providing care is taken to avoid contamination from maternal DNA.

DISORDERS OF CARBOHYDRATE METABOLISM

GALACTOSAEMIA

In classical galactosaemia, deficiency of the enzyme galactose 1-phosphate uridyl transferase (Gal 1-PUT) leads to accumulation of galactose 1-phosphate, galactitol and galactose in all tissues, and to severe liver disease. Basic liver biochemistry tests are usually grossly abnormal with a predominately cholestatic picture but also with raised plasma aminotransferases indicating hepatocellular necrosis. Other frequent laboratory findings include a raised INR, haemolytic anaemia and amino aciduria together with proteinuria indicating renal impairment. The exact mechanism of hepatic toxicity is unknown, but may be related to cellular ATP depletion due to intracellular accumulation of galactose 1-phosphate restricting the availability of phosphate for formation of high energy bonds. This is supported by the absence of liver disease in the majority of patients with epimerase deficiency galactosaemia where uridine diphosphate galactose accumulation occurs to a greater extent than galactose 1-phosphate.

A test for reducing substances (not glucose specific) in urine should, if positive, raise the suspicion of galactosaemia. Thin layer chromatography of urine for sugars will confirm the presence of excess galactose although this is not specific for galactosaemia. The definitive diagnosis of galactosaemia requires demonstration of absent or low Gal 1-PUT activity in erythrocytes.

FRUCTOSAEMIA

Three genetic defects in fructose metabolism have been identified: essential fructosaemia, hereditary fructose intolerance and fructose 1,6-diphosphatase deficiency. The first of these is a benign condition due caused by hepatic fructokinase deficiency. Hereditary fructose intolerance is also predominantly benign providing dietary fructose is avoided. If a high fructose intake is maintained then severe liver and kidney damage can occur. In a manner analogous to galactosaemia, hepatic toxicity in fructosaemia is believed to be due to fructose 1-phosphate accumulation reducing the availability of phosphate for ATP formation. The plasma aminotransferases are markedly elevated with a conjugated hyperbilirubinaemia and raised INR. Other abnormalities include: hypoalbuminaemia, hypokalaemia, hypophosphataemia, a profound hypoglycaemia and thrombocytopenia. The renal damage leads to amino aciduria and proteinuria.

Fructose 1,6-diphosphatase deficiency usually has less severe effects on the liver. Plasma aminotransferase activities are mildly to moderately elevated but, in contrast to hereditary fructose intolerance, plasma bilirubin concentrations are at most only mildly increased. The prominent features are hypoglycaemia, lactic acidaemia, amino acidaemia (particularly alanine and glutamine) and a marked ketoacidosis. The definitive diagnosis of both this disorder and of hereditary fructose intolerance requires demonstration of a deficiency in the respective enzymes in liver biopsy specimens.

GLYCOGEN STORAGE DISEASES

Seven distinct types and several sub-types of inherited disorders of carbohydrate metabolism which lead to abnormal glycogen storage have been identified (Figure 4.7). Type VI includes a number of sub-types of phosphorylase or phosphorylase kinase deficiencies which in some classifications are designated as types IX to XII. Most of these present in childhood and prognosis varies according to the type, from very poor (types II and IV) to good (type VI).

Glycogen storage diseases			
Type	Synonym	Tissues involved	Enzyme defect
Ia	Von Gierke's disease	Liver, kidney, intestine	Glucose-6-phosphatase
Ib		Liver, kidney, intestine	Glucose-6-phosphate transporter
II	Pompe's disease	All tissues	Lysosomal α1,4- and α1,6-glucosidase
III	Cori disease Forbe's disease Limit dextrinosis	Liver, muscle, heart and other tissues	Amylo 1,6-glucosidase ($\pm$)-phosphorylase kinase
IV	Andersen disease Amylopectinosis	Most tissues	Amylo (1,4)-(1,6)-transgluconidase
V	McArdle syndrome	Skeletal muscle only	Muscle phosphorylase
VI	Hers disease	Liver only	Liver phosphorylase
VII	Tauri disease	Skeletal muscle, erythrocytes	Phosphofructokinase

Figure 4.7 The glycogen storage diseases

In the glycogen storage disorders that affect the liver, hypoglycaemia is the most significant finding and may cause significant cerebral damage with severe learning difficulties if frequent or prolonged. The hepatocytes are distended with accumulation of glycogen and excess fat. Cell necrosis results in fibrosis with progression to cirrhosis in patients who survive past childhood. Jaundice is rare and standard liver biochemistry tests may be normal or indicate only mild cholestasis until the later stages when hepatic failure occurs. Other frequent laboratory findings include hyperlipidaemia, acidosis and hyperuricaemia. Clinical management requires knowledge of the type of glycogen storage disease by measurement of the specific enzyme activities in the tissues. Among those that affect the liver, the defects can be identified in peripheral blood leucocytes in type II, III, IV or VI, but liver biopsies are required for types Ia and Ib.

DISORDERS OF AMINO ACID METABOLISM

The only genetically mediated disorder of amino acid metabolism that has so far been identified as a cause of significant liver disease is hereditary tyrosinaemia. Two types of this autosomal recessive condition are recognised, type I which is due to a deficiency of fumarylacetoacetase and is associated with a poor prognosis and type II which is due to the deficiency of the cytosolic enzyme tyrosine amino-transferase and is not associated with liver damage.

Type I tyrosinaemia is rare with an incidence of fewer than 1:100,000. It usually presents in early childhood with vomiting, diarrhoea, hepatosplenomegaly, ascites and failure to thrive. Renal tubular dysfunction and hypophosphataemic rickets may also be present. Death may occur from acute hepatic failure within the first year of life. Those who survive longer succumb to primary liver cancer in the first two decades of life. There is moderate to severe derangement of the standard liver biochemistry tests and a markedly raised INR. The characteristic laboratory finding is a marked amino acidaemia, with tyrosine, phenylalanine and methionine concentrations being particularly elevated. Plasma AFP concentrations are often markedly elevated (up to 100-fold) even in the absence of liver cancer. The diagnostic feature is the finding of succinylacetone in the urine, this being formed from maleylacetoacetate and fumarylacetoacetate (Figure 4.8). High excretion of 5-aminolaevulinate is due to inhibition of porphobilinogen synthase by succinylacetone. It is believed that the hepatic injury is caused by glutathione depletion due to the reaction of reduced glutathione with succinylacetone and its precursors, which accumulates in the liver and kidneys.

The only effective treatment is liver transplantation but recently treatment with 2-(2-nitro-4-trifluro,ethylbenzoyl)-1, 3-cyclohexanedione (NTBC), which inhibits 4-hydroxyphenylpyruvate dioxygenase, has been shown to slow the progression of the disease. Longer term studies will be needed to determine if NTBC is an alternative to liver transplantation in type I tyrosinaemia.

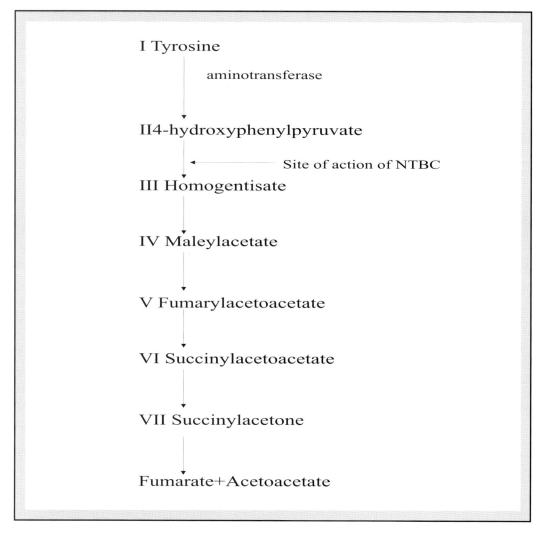

I Tyrosine

aminotransferase

II 4-hydroxyphenylpyruvate

Site of action of NTBC

III Homogentisate

IV Maleylacetate

V Fumarylacetoacetate

VI Succinylacetoacetate

VII Succinylacetone

Fumarate+Acetoacetate

Figure 4.8 Formation of succinyl acetone in tyrosinaemia type 1 and the site of action of NTBC

THE PORPHYRIAS

The porphyrias are a group of inherited disorders of haem metabolism that lead to abnormal production of porphyrinogens or other precursors in the haem synthetic pathway. Most of the porphyrias present with skin lesions associated with photosensitivity and liver disease is associated with some types (Figure 4.9). The extent of liver involvement varies with the type of porphyria and whether the patient already has liver disease of some other type. Correct identification of the type of porphyria is essential as treatment varies and the condition may be exacerbated by exogenous agents, including alcohol and wide range of drugs, which should be avoided. Initial screening tests for urinary δ-aminolevulinic acid (ALA) and porphobilinogen (PBG) can be helpful but separation of porphyrins in urine or faeces using high performance liquid chromatography is necessary to ensure the correct diagnosis is reached. In cases of acute intermittent porphyria (AIP) measurement of PBG deaminase in erythrocytes can be useful. An increased frequency of the CYS 282TYR and HIS63ASP haemochromatosis mutations has been found in most series of patients with porphyria cutanea tarda (PCT) suggesting a link between mild iron overload and abnormal haem biochemistry.

Porphyria			
Type	**Enzyme defect**	**Chromosome**	**Principal laboratory features**
Protoporphyria	Ferrochelatase	18q21.3	High blood and faecal protoporphyria and coproporphyria. Normal urine porphyrins
Acute intermittent porphyria	Porphobilinogen deaminase	24.1-q24.2	High urinary ALA and PBG
Coproporphyria	Coproporphyrinogen oxidase	9	High urinary ALA and PBG and faecal coproporphyrin
Variegate porphyria	Protoporphyrinogen oxidase	14	High urinary ALA and PBG and faecal protoporphyrin
Porphyria cutanea tarda	Uroporphyrinogen decarboxylase	1q34	Normal urinary ALA and PBG. High urinary uro-porphyrin I and copro-porphyrin I. Elevated plasma ferritin and iron

Figure 4.9 Porphyrias affecting the liver

In protoporphyria the basic liver biochemistry tests at presentation usually show a cholestatic pattern but the disease can progress rapidly to acute hepatic failure. Hereditary coproporphyria, variegate porphyria and AIP can be grouped together as they all have an autosomal dominant mode of inheritance and lead to a potential reduction of haem synthesis and overproduction of ALA. Unless there is concomitant liver disease of some other aetiology, standard liver biochemistry tests usually show a modest increase in plasma aminotransferases as the main abnormality. Many patients have dark urine, which may vary in colour from wine-red to brownish (darkening on standing or exposure to sunlight) and which must be distinguished from the orange-brown colour related to hyperbilirubinaemia in other liver disorders. In patients with porphyria cutanea tarda who have active liver disease there is increased deposition of iron in the liver and a raised plasma ferritin. The results of plasma liver biochemistry tests are also similar to those encountered in haemochromatosis. It is important to note that secondary porphyrinuria with normal ALA or PBG excretion can occur in a wide range of hepatic and non-hepatic disorders including the hereditary conjugated hyperbilirubinaemias.

THE HEREDITARY HYPERBILIRUBINAEMIAS

With the exception of Gilbert's syndrome, the congenital hyperbilirubinaemias are rare conditions and a raised plasma bilirubin is often the only abnormality (Figure 4.10). The congenital hyperbilirubinaemias are conventionally divided into conjugated and unconjugated types, the latter being defined when less than 20% of an elevated bilirubin concentration is in the conjugated state.

HEREDITARY CONJUGATED HYPERBILIRUBINAEMIAS

There are two inherited conjugated hyperbilirubinaemias: Dubin-Johnson syndrome and Rotor's syndrome. Dubin-Johnson syndrome is relatively rare throughout the world, but is commonest in Arab races and in both Ashkenazic and Sephardic Jews. The hyperbilirubinaemia is intermittent and is mixed i.e., conjugated and unconjugated. Examination of the liver reveals lysosomal deposits of a yellow-brown or black melanin-like pigment in hepatocytes. Patients are usually asymptomatic, the condition being identified by mild jaundice on routine screening. Occasionally, pregnancy or oral contraception may unmask the condition. Standard liver biochemistry tests are typically normal. Urinary excretion of urobilinogen and coproporphyrin I are increased, and that of coproporphyrin III is decreased.

Rotor's syndrome was first identified in the Philippine population but appears to have a world-wide distribution. As with Dubin-Johnson syndrome, the hyperbilirubinaemia may fluctuate with conjugated bilirubin concentrations being higher than unconjugated. Other liver biochemistry tests are usually normal. The urinary excretion of coproporphyrin is increased due to increases in both the I and III isomers, which can be used to differentiate Rotor's syndrome from Dubin-

Johnson syndrome in which there is a disproportionate increase in isomer I.

Congenital hyperbilirubinaemias				
	Gilbert's syndrome	Crigler-Najjar syndrome Type 1	Type 2	Dubin-Johnson syndrome	Rotor's syndrome
Incidence	Common	Rare	Rare	Uncommon	Rare
Mode of inheritance	Autosomal dominant	Autosomal recessive	?	Autosomal recessive	Autosomal recessive
Clinical features other than jaundice	None	Kernicterus; death in infancy	Usually none	None	None
Plasma bilirubin (μmol/L)	Variable normal to 100	300 - 600	100 - 400	Variable 35 - 100	Variable 35 - 100
Age of onset	Any usually adolescence	First 10 days of life	First year of life	Early adult	Childhood

Figure 4.10 Features of the congenital hyperbilirubinaemias

HEREDITARY UNCONJUGATED HYPERBILIRUBINAEMIAS
The hereditary unconjugated hyperbilirubinaemias comprise the benign, relatively common Gilbert's syndrome and the rare Crigler-Najjar syndrome, of which there are two types. Type 1 Crigler-Najjar syndrome is inherited in an autosomal recessive manner and is due to an absence of UDP-glucuronosyl transferase. Presentation is within 48 hours of birth and the jaundice rapidly escalates to a degree that results in kernicterus if treatment is not rapidly instituted. In the past the condition was invariably fatal within the first year of life but liver transplantation has been used successfully to treat the condition. Type 2 Crigler-Najjar syndrome is less severe and the jaundice may occur later in life.

In contrast, Gilbert's syndrome is an entirely benign condition which is characterised by asymptomatic episodes of mild to moderate (up to 80-100 μmol/L) hyperbilirubinaemia. All other biochemical liver tests are normal and histology reveals no evidence of liver damage. It usually first becomes apparent in early adulthood either during a routine health check or because the individual is noted to be slightly jaundiced. The jaundice tends to be more pronounced when the affected person is tired, or has been fasting or has an intercurrent illness such as influenza. It is a common condition which is estimated to affect up to 7% of the population and is seen more often in males than females. The molecular basis of Gilbert's syndrome has now been elucidated and results from a reduction in the concentration of the isoform of UDP-glucuronosyl transferase responsible for bilirubin conjugation (UGT-1A). UGT-1A is encoded by the UDG gene family which is composed of multiple unique forms of exon 1, each specific for one isoenzyme, and four common exons. The most common mutation in the UGT-1A gene is a TA insertion in the repetitive TATA-box of the gene promoter. The mutation reduces the expression of this gene and homozygosity results in the inability to produce sufficient UGT-1A to respond to increases in demand for bilirubin conjugation.The importance of the condition lies in its recognition, so that the individual is spared intensive investigations. Following a single intravenous dose of 50 mg of nicotinic acid, there is a 2-3 fold increase in unconjugated plasma bilirubin over the next three hours. In unaffected individuals, or in those with haemolytic jaundice, the bilirubin concentration may increase slightly but does not double. However, this test is not widely used because some authorities doubt its specificity and the nicotinic acid makes the subject feel unwell. A similar increase in plasma bilirubin occurs in subjects with Gilbert's syndrome following prolonged fasting (48 hours) and this can be used as an alternative to the nicotinic acid test.

MISCELLANEOUS CONDITIONS AFFECTING THE LIVER

In addition to those covered already, there are numerous other disorders of the liver in which genetic factors, or at least a genetic susceptibility to external agents, have been identified or are suspected. Some of these conditions are due to primary metabolic defects and others are secondary to anatomical abnormalities. Some present in early infancy and form part of the differential diagnosis of neonatal hepatitis, whilst others may present much later with cirrhosis.

CONGENITAL HEPATIC FIBROSIS

This condition is defined pathologically as the presence of bands of fibrous tissue joining portal tracts in the liver and often containing spaces lined by bile ducts. Portal hypertension is the major feature and the condition is often associated with renal disorders such as infantile polycystic disease. As in polycystic disease of the liver and kidneys, hepatocellular function seems not to be compromised and mild to moderate elevation of alkaline phosphatase (and occasionally GGT) is often the only plasma biochemical liver abnormality detected. The disorder must be distinguished from other forms of cirrhosis, usually on the basis of clinical findings and liver histopathology.

INTRAHEPATIC BILIARY HYPOPLASIA (ALAGILLE'S SYNDROME)
Alagille's syndrome is a rare condition (estimated incidence one per 100,000 live births) characterized by an absence or paucity of interlobular bile ducts associated with a range of cardiovascular, skeletal, facial and ocular anomalies. The aetiology of the condition is unknown but a number of familial cases have been reported suggesting a genetic defect. In a proportion of cases a partial deletion of chromosome 20 has been observed. The absence of bile ductules leads to retention of bile in the hepatocytes and in time to a clinical picture of chronic cholestasis. Most cases present in early childhood with a conjugated hyperbilirubinaemia and a hepatitic type of illness. The aminotransferases, alkaline phosphatase and GGT are markedly raised, to up to 30 times the reference interval. Vitamin K malabsorption may lead to spontaneous bleeding. Plasma cholesterol and triglycerides are raised in up to 80% of cases with values up to three times the reference interval for children being common. The chronic hypercholesterolaemia results in xanthelasma in many children with Alagille's syndrome. The association of cholestatic liver disease in infancy with cardiac abnormalities should lead to a consideration of Alagille's syndrome.

BYLER'S DISEASE
This severe intrahepatic cholestatic disorder was first described in several members of an Amish family named Byler. Onset is usually within the first year of life but jaundice may be intermittent initially, becoming persistent later. The standard liver biochemistry tests are severely deranged with elevated plasma aminotransferase activities, indicating hepatocellular necrosis, in addition to hyperbilirubinaemia. This contrasts with the similar, but generally milder, condition known as benign recurrent intrahepatic cholestasis. Both are inherited in an autosomal recessive mode and are thought to be manifestations of two different mutations on a gene on chromosome 18q 21-22.

CYSTIC FIBROSIS.
Hepatobiliary abnormalities of varying severity are a fairly common and well-recognised complication of cystic fibrosis (CF). Excessive accumulation of lipid can be seen in hepatocytes but does not necessarily have major consequences. Occasionally, a prolonged conjugated hyperbilirubinaemia (due to extrahepatic biliary obstruction) together with severe hypoalbuminaemia is seen in infants with CF. As these children progress to adolescence, up to 20% may develop a biliary-

type cirrhosis. Since the discovery of the gene responsible for CF, many different mutations have been reported. Not all children with CF develop liver disease and those that do may represent a distinct phenotypic variant of the disease. Initial impressions are that liver disease is less common in patients homozygous for the common Δ508 mutation and more common when other mutations are present either heterozygous with Δ508 or as homozygotes. Studies are underway to determine if there is a correlation between the disease phenotype and the genotype.

MITOCHONDRIAL DISORDERS OF FATTY ACID METABOLISM

Several disorders involving fatty acid oxidation can present with hepatomegaly and symptoms resembling those seen in Reye's syndrome e.g., hyperammonaemia, hypoglycaemia, etc. Long chain acyl-CoA dehydrogenase deficiency produces a syndrome in which non-ketotic hypoglycaemia, dicarboxylic aciduria and low tissue and plasma carnitine concentrations are the principal biochemical findings. Patients usually present in childhood and may have cardiomyopathy as well as hepatomegaly. A similar picture but with earlier onset (as early as 9 weeks of age) has been described for systemic carnitine deficiency. Initial symptoms are vomiting with lethargy which can progress quickly to coma. Standard liver biochemistry tests are abnormal with a pattern similar to that seen in Reye's syndrome. A further condition, carnitine palmityl transferase deficiency, has also been reported to present with hepatomegaly.

DISORDERS OF LYSOSOMAL ENZYMES

Almost all disorders of lysosomal enzymes are the result of the absence of specific enzymes which degrade complex macromolecules. Although most of these disorders feature multi-system symptomatology with neurological defects particularly prominent, hepatosplenomegaly is a common finding. The lipidoses and mucopolysaccharidoses are the two groups with a high prevalence of hepatic involvement.

The most significant group of the lipidoses that cause hepatic damage are the sphingomyelin-cholesterol lipidoses or Niemann-Pick diseases. In Niemann-Pick type II disease there is a defect in the translocation of exogenous cholesterol in lysosomes. More than half the patients with Niemann-Pick type II disease present in early infancy with jaundice as part of a hepatitic syndrome. Around one third of patients die of liver disease in the first 6 months of life but in those who survive, the features of hepatitis regress and although some degree of hepatomegaly may persist symptomatic liver disease is rare. In acid esterase deficiency (Wolman's disease) and hepatic cholesterol ester storage disease there is excessive accumulation of cholesterol esters and triglycerides in many organs, particularly the liver. Standard liver biochemistry tests are usually abnormal with hypercholesterolaemia and hypertriglyceridaemia in the majority.

At least seven types of mucopolysaccharide storage disorders have been identified. The diseases are associated with characteristic facies and hepatosplenomegaly is a common feature. Basic liver biochemistry tests show mild to moderate non-specific abnormalities. Diagnosis is based on the pattern of excretion of dermatan, heparin or keratin sulphates and assay of the specific enzymes in leucocytes.

DISORDERS OF PEROXISOMAL FUNCTION

Over the past decade knowledge of peroxisomal function and the peroxisomal disorders has expanded enormously. Zellweger's syndrome is the most common of these disorders with liver involvement but adrenoleucodystrophy, Refsum disease and pipecolic acidaemia can also involve the liver. Zellweger's syndrome is characterized by the absence of peroxisomes and presents with severe neurological deficits from birth. Hepatomegaly is present at birth in a proportion of patients but is almost universal by 2 months of age. Standard liver biochemistry tests are abnormal and hypoglycaemia may be present. There are characteristic abnormalities of bile acid synthesis and accumulation of very long chain fatty acids, phytanic acid and pipecolic acid (a product of lysine degradation).

DEFECTS IN BILE SALT METABOLISM

Bile salt synthesis occurs in the mitochondria and peroxisomes of the liver and involves more than 15 enzymes and 29 intermediates. Deficiency of primary bile acids reduces bile production and flow leading to malabsorption, while some of the intermediary metabolites may have some toxicity to hepatocytes. Two distinct inborn errors of bile acid metabolism associated with liver disease have been identified; 3β-hydroxy-Δ-5 C27 steroid dehydrogenase deficiency and 3-oxo-Δ^4-steroid β-reductase deficiency. Characteristic patterns of bile acids in urine or plasma can be identified using GC-MS analysis of bile acids.

UREA CYCLE DISORDERS

Inherited deficiencies of all four of the enzymes of the urea cycle are known, carbamyl phosphate synthetase (CPSD), ornithine transcarbamylase (OTCD), arginosuccinic acid synthetase (ASD) and arginosuccinate lyase (ALD), and can be associated with liver disease. There is a considerable variation in clinical presentation with some cases presenting in the neonatal period and others having no symptoms until puberty. Hyperammonaemia is a characteristic feature of urea cycle defects, whilst hepatomegaly and raised plasma aminotransferases indicates hepatic involvement. Plasma glutamine is markedly raised in patients with hyperammonaemia coma. The excess ammonia and glutamate damage astrocytes in the central nervous system leading to cerebral oedema and can also cause hepatocyte necrosis leading to progressive fibrosis and cirrhosis. Orotic acid, formed from diversion of carbamyl phosphate to pyrimidine, can be detected in urine in OTCD,

ASD and ALD deficiencies. Measurement of plasma ornithine, citrulline and arginosuccinic acid will define the disorder in most cases, but confirmation by measuring the specific enzyme in liver biopsy for CPSD and OTCD or in fibroblasts for ASD and ALD should be undertaken.

FURTHER READING

Adams PC, Valberg LS. Evolving expression of hereditary haemochromatosis. Semin Liv Dis 1996; **16:** 47-54

Baker A, Gormally S, Saxena R, Baldwin D, Drumm B, Bonham J, Portmann B, Mowat AP. Copper associated liver disease in childhood. J Hepatol 1995; **23:** 538-43.

Clayton PT. Inborn errors of bile acid metabolism. J Inher Metab Dis 1991; **14:** 478-96.

Da Costa CM, Baldwin D, Portmann B, Lolin Y, Mowat AP, Mieli-Vergani G. Value of urinary copper excretion after penicillamine challenge in the diagnosis of Wilson's disease. Hepatology 1992; **15:** 609-15.

Knisely AS. Iron and paediatric liver disease. Semin Liv Dis 1994; **14:** 229-35.

Krittigen EA. Tyrosinaemia type I - an update. J Inher Metab Dis 1992; **14:** 554-62.

Lindstedt S, Holme E, Lock EA, Hjalamrson O, Strandvik B, Treatment of hereditary tyrosinaemia type I by inhibition of 4-hydroxyphenylpyruvate dioxygenase. Lancet 1992; **340:** 813-7.

Mowat AP. Liver disorders in childhood. 3rd edn. London: Butterworths, 1994.

Norman MR, Mowat AP, Hutchinson DCS. Molecular basis, clinical consequences and diagnosis of alpha-1-antitrypsin deficiency. Ann Clin Biochem 1997; **34:** 230-45.

Rank JM, Straka JG, Bloomer JR. Liver in disorders of porphyrin metabolism. J Gastroenterol Hepatol 1990; **5:** 573-85.

Schilsky ML. Wilson disease: Genetic basis of copper toxicity and natural history. Semin Liv Dis 1996; **16:** 83-95.

Shin YS. The diagnosis of glycogen storage disease. J Inher Metab Dis 1990; **13:** 419-34.

Teckman J, Perlmutter DH. Conceptual advances in the pathogenesis and treatment of childhood metabolic liver disease. Gastroenterol 1995; **108:** 1263-79.

Van Berge Heneguwen GP. Benign recurrent intrahepatic cholestasis and Byler's disease: one gene, two diseases? J Hepatol 1996; **25:** 395-7.

Chapter 5.

Xenobiotic-induced liver disease

GENERAL ASPECTS OF DRUG-INDUCED LIVER DISEASE

The liver is the first solid organ to come into contact with ingested agents and is the main site of metabolism of most drugs and other potentially toxic substances. Its central role in the biotransformation of xenobiotics is probably the most important factor in rendering it susceptible to damage by such agents. Individual susceptibility to hepatic injury by a particular drug or other toxin is influenced by many factors, including genetic predisposition, age, gender, nutritional status, pre-existing disease(s) and interaction with other drugs.

More than 600 drugs or other chemical agents have been implicated as causative agents of liver damage and the list continues to grow year by year. Drug-induced hepatic injury is estimated to account for about 10% of all liver disease in adults worldwide and the prevalence increases with age. To cover adequately all of the agents known to exhibit some degree of hepatotoxicity is beyond the scope of this book and this chapter is intended only as an aide mémoire to the possibility that abnormal biochemical liver tests may be drug-related. Liver damage due to alcohol and paracetamol is covered in some detail because these are the two most commonly encountered agents in general laboratory and clinical medicine.

THE SPECTRUM OF DRUG-INDUCED LIVER DISEASE

Drug-induced liver disease can encompass virtually all known forms of hepatic injury, both acute and chronic. Liver damage may be the only effect of the drug or there may be systemic manifestations. The timescale for development of hepatic lesions can vary from days or weeks to several months and depends partly on whether the agent is a 'predictable' or an 'idiosyncratic' hepatotoxin. A 'predictable' hepatotoxin is one which has an intrinsic hepatotoxicity and, in the case of a drug, is usually safe at normal therapeutic doses but exhibits dose-dependent toxicity if these doses are exceeded. An 'idiosyncratic' toxin causes liver damage in only a small proportion of exposed individuals in a manner which is seldom dose-dependent and is often not reproducible in animal models. With the latter, the hepatic injury may be accompanied by symptoms of generalised hypersensitivity such as fever, rashes and eosinophilia.

In many cases of drug-induced hepatotoxicity there are no clinical manifestations and liver damage is detected only by elevated plasma enzyme activities. These minor abnormalities are often transient, even if therapy is continued. From the diagnostic standpoint, induction of gamma-glutamyl transferase (GGT) is relatively common, which reduces the value of this test for liver disease. However, persisting or increasing elevations of plasma enzymes often signals overt hepatic injury and may warrant withdrawal of the drug.

It must be remembered that many drugs induce the synthesis of enzymes involved in their own metabolism. From the point of view of toxicity, this can be either advantageous or disadvantageous. If the parent compound is toxic, enzyme induction can hasten clearance to non-toxic metabolites. Conversely, if the metabolite is toxic, enzyme induction may result in increased toxicity. Additionally, some drugs are metabolised via two or more different pathways and alterations in the balance between induction or deficiencies of the enzymes involved in the different pathways can influence the toxicity of the drug.

Drug-induced hepatic damage may be either hepatocellular (i.e., with liver cell necrosis and/or steatosis), or cholestatic (i.e., leading to reduced bile flow and jaundice but little parenchymal damage), or of a mixed type with simultaneous features of parenchymal and cholestatic injury. Examples of drugs that cause these different patterns of liver damage are given in Figures 5.1 and 5.2. These lists are not exhaustive but they illustrate the range of drugs in routine clinical use that can be hepatotoxic.

The clinical and biochemical features of acute drug-induced hepatocellular injury can resemble those of acute viral hepatitis. The plasma aminotransferase activities rise sharply and can reach values more than 100-fold greater than normal, whereas plasma alkaline phosphatase activity seldom rises more than 3-fold. A rise in bilirubin concentration tends not to occur until severe hepatic necrosis is present and is a poor prognostic sign, indicating impending acute liver failure (see Chapter 1). Where steatosis is the major feature, the clinical and biochemical manifestations resemble those of acute fatty liver of pregnancy or of Reye's syndrome. Paracetamol is probably the best known predictably hepatotoxic drug that in overdose leads to parenchymal liver damage, but other relatively frequently used drugs (e.g., valproate, methyldopa, phenytoin, etc.) can also cause hepatocellular necrosis of sufficient severity to lead to acute liver failure, as can several plant toxins - of which that produced by the poisonous mushroom Amanita phalloides is perhaps the best known example.

Chronic liver damage resembling autoimmune hepatitis (see Chapter 6), with hypergammaglobulinaemia and circulating autoantibodies, can be produced idiosyncratically by a number of drugs including methyldopa and the antibiotic minocycline. Phospholipidosis, characterised by engorgement of lysosomes with

Drugs causing hepatocellular injury	
Analgesics	Dantrolene
	Gold (m)
	Paracetamol
	Salicylates
Anaesthetics	Enflurane
	Halothane
Anticonvulsants	Phenytoin
	Valproate
Antimicrobials	Antimonials
	Clindamycin
	Didanosine
	Ketoconazole
	Rifampicin
	Sulphonamides (m)
	Minocyline
Antineoplastic	Etoposide
	Fluorouracil
	Methotrexate
	Vincristine
Cardiovascular drugs	Amiodarone
	Diltiazem
	Methyldopa
	Perhexiline
	Procainamide (m)
	Tycrinafin
Endocrine agents	Propylthiouracil
	Tamoxifen
Psychotropic drugs	Clozapine
	Maprotiline
	Tricyclics (m)
Miscellaneous	Disulfiram
	Vitamin A
	Ecstasy

Figure 5.1 Examples of drugs that can cause a predominantly hepatocellular pattern of liver injury (m = mixed pattern)

Drugs causing cholestatic injury	
Analgesics	Naproxen Penicillamine Propoxyphene
Antimicrobials	Cephalosporins Erythromycin esters Sulphonamides (m) Zidovudine
Antineoplastics	Azathioprine
Cardiovascular drugs	Ajmaline (m) Captopril Enalapril Pheninolane (m) Thiazides (m)
Endocrine agents	Carbimazole Methimazole (m) Oral contraceptives (m) Thiouracil
Psychotropic drugs	Chlordiazepoxide Diazepam Haloperidol Mianserin Trimipramine (m) Tricyclics (some)
Miscellaneous	Cimetidine Ranitidine

Figure 5.2. Examples of drugs that can cause a predominantly cholestatic hepatic injury. (m= mixed pattern)

phospholipids, is seen with the cardiovascular drugs perhexiline and amiodarone. This is often accompanied by steatosis and cirrhosis with histological features of alcoholic liver disease. Chronic cholestatic drug-induced syndromes can mimic primary biliary cirrhosis (see Chapter 6). Hepatic adenomas and veno-occlusive and granulomatous diseases may also occur as a consequence of chronic drug therapy.

MECHANISMS OF CHEMICAL HEPATOTOXICITY

The biochemical reactions involved in drug metabolism by the liver lead to detoxification through conversion of the relatively non-polar (lipid-soluble) compounds to more polar (water-soluble) substances that can be excreted in the bile or urine. These reactions are catalysed by a large number of enzymes, but the most important quantitatively are those comprising the mixed-function oxidase system. Most of the drug metabolising enzymes exist as families of isoenzymes (e.g., the cytochrome P450 group), each having discrete but overlapping substrate specificities and capable of handling a broad range of both xenobiotics and endogenous compounds. Thus competition between endogenous substances and drugs can lead to toxicity. The same pathways can sometimes lead to production of reactive metabolites which readily bind to various cellular macromolecules such as nucleic acids and proteins, and can thereby cause cellular changes that may lead to cell death.

Each of the enzymes involved in drug metabolising is under homeostatic control influenced by genetic and environmental factors. Several of these systems are reduced in activity in neonates and sometimes also in the elderly, which can lead to direct toxicity through the pharmacological effects of certain drugs. Other factors that can diminish enzyme activity, and thereby enhance direct heptotoxicity, include malnutrition (especially protein deficiency) and severe disease. This is particularly true in patients with pre-existing liver disease, in which the reduction in synthetic function (with consequent hypoalbuminaemia, leading to reduction in protein binding and increased concentrations of free drug in the circulation), and extrahepatic shunting can profoundly affect the hepatotoxicity of xenobiotics.

GENETIC PREDISPOSITION TO DRUG HEPATOTOXICITY

It is now clear that genetic predispositions underlie some idiosyncratic drug hepatotoxic reactions. Genetic polymorphisms in drug metabolising enzymes can lead to alterations (enhancements or reductions) in pathways of metabolism of the drugs, and have been shown to be at least partly responsible for the hepatotoxicity of perhexiline dihydralazine and the sulphonamides (Figure 5.3). Other polymorphisms have been postulated in sulphoxidation and glutathione synthesis but have yet to be confirmed. A few of the more extensively studied polymorphisms are discussed below by way of illustration.

CYTOCHROME P450 2D6 (DEBRISOQUINE) POLYMORPHISM

Genetic polymorphism of the cytochrome P450 2D6 (CYP 2D6) subfamily of enzymes is associated with deficiency of debrisoquine/dextromethorphan oxidation. This deficiency occurs in 5-10% of the European population. Most patients with perhexiline-induced liver injury have been found to be poor metabolisers of the drug and it is believed that excessive accumulation of perhexiline in hepatocytes leads to the phospholipidosis that is typically seen in these cases. The original phenotyping method using a test dose of debrisoquine has largely been replaced by genotyping. The gene for CYP 2D6 is on chromosome 22 and nine mutant alleles have been identified. The most common mutant allele is CYP 2D6B, accounting for over 70% of all null alleles, with CYP 2D6A and CYP 2D6D (deletion allele) accounting for most of the remainder. It has been suggested that chlorpromazine hepatotoxicity may be more common in individuals with a high debrisoquine oxidation capacity but this awaits confirmation.

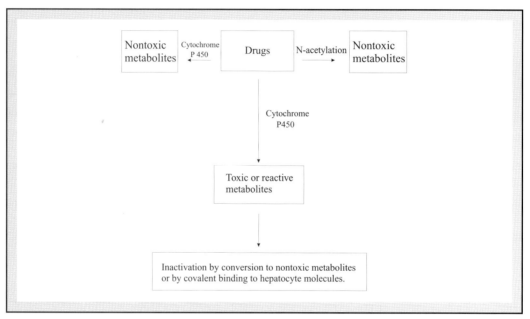

Figure 5.3 Genetic polymorphism in drug metabolising enzymes

N-ACETYLATION

Polymorphism in N-acetylation was first described with respect to isoniazid metabolism over 30 years ago. Virtually all cases of sulphonamide and dihydralazine hepatotoxicity have occurred in subjects who are homozygous for a defective N-acetyltransferase 2 (NAT2) gene and are consequently slow acetylators. In such individuals metabolism of these drugs is shifted to the cytochrome P450 pathways, leading to production of reactive metabolites: hydroxylamines from sulphonamides and free radicals from dihydralazine. The use of test doses of a drug (caffeine or dapsone) to phenotype acetylation status has largely been replaced by genotyping methods. Eight mutant alleles in the NAT2 gene have now been described in Caucasian and Asian subjects, six of which code for the slow acetylation phenotype which has a prevalence of up to 70% in some populations. As hepatotoxicity is not invariable with these drugs, other factors must also play a role in the development of hepatic injury.

AZATHIOPRINE METABOLISM

Azathioprine is widely used as an immunosuppressive agent in organ transplantation and for treatment of autoimmune diseases, and as a cytotoxic agent in certain malignant conditions. It is normally first converted non-enzymatically in the blood to 6-mercaptopurine, which is then further metabolised via two main pathways: i) conversion by hypoxanthine-guanine phosphoribosyl transferase to 6-thioguanine nucleotides (6-TGNs), the active metabolites that exert the immunosuppressive and cytotoxic effects of the drug, and ii) conversion to inactive metabolites through the action of thiopurine methyltransferase (TPMT), synthesis of which is inducible by azathioprine. The efficacy of the drug and the frequency of adverse side-effects (notably myelosuppression) vary widely between individuals. It is now known that this is due to genetic polymorphisms determining TPMT activity. About 1 in 300 individuals in the population are homozygous for one or more alleles that encode an inactive form of TPMT and about 11% are heterozygous. Such individuals have very low TPMT activities and, consequently, most of the drug is converted to the highly toxic 6-TGNs. They require much lower doses of the drug to achieve the desired therapeutic effects and suffer much more frequently from adverse side-effects at standard doses. Conversely, other alleles appear to encode particularly active forms of TPMT or are much more sensitive to induction of the enzyme by azathioprine, leading to rapid conversion of the drug to inactive metabolites. Individuals with these alleles are much more tolerant of the drug and require higher doses for therapeutic effect. Screening for these polymorphisms is currently done by measuring TPMT activity in erythrocytes but it is likely that genotyping techniques will soon be developed.

ALCOHOL-RELATED LIVER DISEASE

Moderate consumption of alcohol in a social setting is considered by many to be a normal part of everyday life. However, in excess, alcohol has an intrinsic hepatotoxicity. Episodic bouts of heavy drinking (> 300g ethanol/day) may sometimes lead to acute alcoholic hepatitis but, if interspersed by periods of abstinence, may not result in chronic liver disease. Rather, it is the total amount of alcohol consumed together with the duration of drinking and individual susceptibility that determine whether (and to what degree) the liver will be damaged. The form in which alcohol is consumed (beer, wine, spirits, etc.) is largely irrelevant. However, the higher the alcohol content of the beverage the lower the fluid volume that needs to be consumed before a harmful level of intake is reached (Figure 5.4). There is evidence that a moderate daily alcohol intake (15-30 g/day) may have beneficial effects on the cardiovascular system and seldom leads to liver damage, although this is still slightly controversial.

Alcohol content of beverages			
Beverage	**% alcohol (v/v)**	**Measure**	**Ethanol content (g)**
Beer	4	per pint (560 mL)	25
Table wine	12	per glass (125 mL) per bottle (750 mL)	15 90
Fortified wines (sherry, port etc.)	20	per glass (75 mL) per bottle (750 mL)	15 150
Spirits (whiskey, gin etc.)	37.5	per measure (25 mL) per bottle (750 mL)	19 280
Liqueurs	27.5	per glass (60 mL) per bottle (750 mL)	16 200

Figure 5.4 The approximate alcohol content of common alcoholic beverages

The risk of developing cirrhosis increases about 5-fold at an intake of 50 g/day and is more than 25-fold when intake exceeds 100 g/day. Women appear to be more susceptible to alcohol-related liver damage than men, even when differences in body weight are taken into account, and tend to develop cirrhosis at lower daily alcohol intakes over shorter periods. This may be due partly to the higher body fat/weight ratio in women compared to men and partly to hormonal differences. However, the fact that some individuals can consume fairly large amounts of alcohol over many years without any significant liver injury, while others develop cirrhosis after much shorter periods on lower alcohol intakes, suggests that other factors defining individual susceptibility are involved.

Histologically, three forms of alcohol-related liver damage are recognised: steatosis (fatty liver), hepatitis and fibrosis/cirrhosis. Features of each may be found alone or in combination with the others and the clinical and laboratory findings, as well as prognosis, will depend on the existence (or co-existence) of these features (Figure 5.5). Although normal or near-normal liver architecture may be found in individuals consuming excessive amounts of alcohol, most heavy drinkers will have some degree of fat deposition in their livers. Fatty liver is the most benign of the alcohol-induced changes and is often reversible by avoiding alcohol. In its more severe forms, the fatty change may be accompanied by fibrous tissue deposition (possibly leading to cirrhosis), but occasionally, large fat vacuoles may rupture hepatocytes and the ensuing inflammatory reaction can lead to formation of lipogranulomas.

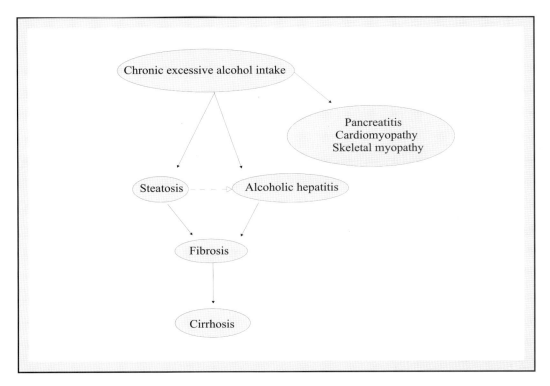

Figure 5.5 Stages in the development of alcoholic liver disease

Alcoholic hepatitis can present acutely or be insidious. The histological features include foci of (usually centrilobular) necrosis with spidery fibrosis, leucocytic infiltration (predominantly polymorphs) and cytoplasmic inclusions of a granular material known as Mallory's hyaline. Although strongly suggestive of alcohol-induced liver damage, Mallory's hyaline can also be seen in cirrhosis of other aetiologies. Alcoholic hepatitis may resolve upon cessation of drinking but it is generally associated with a high mortality, particularly when renal failure supervenes, with 30-50% of patients dying within four weeks of hospitalisation.

The precise mechanisms that lead to the various forms of alcohol-induced liver damage are poorly understood. Approximately 80% of any alcohol ingested is metabolised by the liver and 10% by other tissues, the remainder being excreted unchanged. Ethanol is initially converted to acetaldehyde by various enzymes, including the mixed function oxidase system, but alcohol dehydrogenase (ADH) is quantitatively the most important. The acetaldehyde is then converted to acetate by aldehyde dehydrogenase (ALDH). There are marked genetic polymorphisms in ADH and ALDH, which may account for the variability in susceptibility to liver damage between individuals who consume large amounts of alcohol. At each of these two initial steps in the metabolism of ethanol, NADH is generated and its increased availability promotes formation of lipids, ketones, lactate and porphyrinogens. This leads to fat deposition in hepatocytes, as well as hyperlipi-daemia, ketosis, lactic acidaemia and porphyrinuria. Although ethanol itself may cause liver injury, it is more likely that acetaldehyde (being a more reactive compound) is the primary hepatotoxin. Acetaldehyde can inhibit cellular respiration and may be involved in the generation of free radicals, thereby promoting peroxidation of membrane lipids. It can also bind covalently to macromolecules, including haemoglobin, forming adducts which can impair the function of these molecules and/or render them abnormally immunogenic. This may explain the apparent immunological involvement in the persistence of the inflammatory response in alcoholic hepatitis after cessation of drinking in some individuals.

NON-ALCOHOLIC STEATOHEPATITIS

Non-alcoholic steatohepatitis (NASH) is an idiopathic fatty disorder of the liver. It was previously thought to be a rare and relatively benign condition which developed mainly in middle aged females in association with obesity, insulin resistant diabetes and hypertriglyceridaemia. However, increasing awareness of the syndrome during the past decade has led to the recognition that it also occurs in males and can present at almost any age and in many additional settings, including exposure to a wide range of drugs and other hepatotoxins (e.g., occupational exposure to petrochemicals). It is also now known to progress to cirrhosis in some cases and to recur after liver transplantation. There are no specific diagnostic biochemical or serological markers. Biochemical liver tests are mildly or moderately abnormal and occasionally patients have low titres of autoantibodies, which may lead to a misdiagnosis of autoimmune liver disease. A careful history to exclude excessive alcohol intake is essential, but liver biopsy remains the "gold standard" for diagnosis. Typical histological features include micro- and macrovesicular steatosis, mild to moderate portal and lobular inflammation (often with small clusters of polymorphs), liver cell ballooning and perisinusoidal fibrosis. Mallory's hyaline (associated with alcoholic liver disease) may be seen but is often absent and, even in severe cases, the morphological features of severe alcoholic hepatitis such as sclerosing hyaline necrosis are not evident.

DIAGNOSIS OF ALCOHOL-RELATED LIVER DISEASE

When confronted with a patient with signs and symptoms of liver disease who may be misusing alcohol, the clinician needs to address three questions: is the patient actually misusing alcohol; how severe is the liver disease, and is it related to alcohol or is there some other cause? The last question is of particular relevance because it has been suggested that alcohol abusers may have a higher incidence of non alcohol-related liver disease (e.g., chronic viral hepatitis) than the general population.

If there is a clinical suspicion that a patient may be misusing alcohol, a careful drinking history needs to be obtained. This can be difficult to determine accurately because self-denial of alcohol misuse and under-reporting of alcohol consumption are common. Measurement of blood alcohol concentration is not particularly useful in this situation. The half-life of alcohol in the circulation is short and blood alcohol measurements only detect consumption within a 6-8 hour period prior to testing and, in the primary care setting, patients often abstain for a period before their appointment. Urinary alcohol measurements can extend the window of detection to 12-24 hours after consumption but are used much less frequently. A number of other laboratory tests may be useful but their sensitivities and specificities for detection of alcohol misuse varies depending on the population studied (Figure 5.6).

Biochemical tests for alcohol misuse			
Test	Sensitivity in known alcoholic (% range)	Sensitivity in screening programmes (% range)	Specificity (% range)
GGT	60 - 90	20 - 50	55 - 100
MCV	40 - 50	20 - 30	65 - 100
AST	35 - 50	10 - 30	90 - 100
ALT	20 - 50	10 - 30	90 - 100
CDT	65 - 95	20 - 60	90 - 100

Figure 5.6 Sensitivity and specificity of biochemical tests for the detection of alcohol misuse (from Tredger and Sherwood, Annals of Clinical Biochemistry 1997, with permission)

STANDARD BIOCHEMICAL TESTS

The overlapping features and broad spectrum of alcohol-induced liver damage, together with the wide individual variability to excessive alcohol intake, makes the laboratory diagnosis of alcoholic liver disease difficult, and the presence and severity of tissue injury can really only be properly assessed by histological examination of a liver biopsy. Standard laboratory tests can, however, serve as a useful pointer in diagnosis (Figure 5.7). At the outset, it is important to exclude the possibility of non alcohol-related liver diseases that can produce a similar clinical picture, such as viral hepatitis, autoimmune disorders, hereditary haemochromatosis and Wilson disease, by appropriate investigations.

Laboratory results in alcoholic liver disease	
Biochemistry	
GGT	Raised out of proportion to other liver biochemistry tests
AST:ALT ratio	> 2:1
Triglycerides	Increased in fasting state
HDL-cholesterol	Increased
Haematology	
ESR	Raised
MCV	Raised
B12 or folate	Either or both decreased
Immunology	
IgA	Increased with slightly raised IgG and normal IgM
Urinalysis	
Coproporphyrins	Increased

Figure 5.7 Laboratory findings suggestive of alcohol related liver disease

An elevated plasma GGT activity in isolation in a heavy drinker is probably indicative of the mild reversible changes seen in alcoholic steatosis. However, it must be remembered that GGT is highly inducible by a wide range of xenobiotics and the specificity of this test is compromised in patients on drug therapy. In alcoholic hepatitis, the standard biochemical liver tests are almost always deranged but often only moderately. Thus, plasma bilirubin and alkaline phosphatase (ALP) may be normal or only mildly elevated although an increasing bilirubin is associated with a poor prognosis The plasma aminotransferases (AST and ALT) are rarely more than 2-4 times upper normal limits and indeed, an AST greater than 500 IU/L is extremely unusual and is suggestive of another cause. However, the AST is usually increased to a greater degree than the ALT, and it has been proposed that a ratio of AST:ALT of more than 2 is a useful indicator of alcohol-induced liver damage. It is thought that this reflects both pyridoxal 5-phosphate depletion and release of mitochondrial AST (m-AST) from both the liver and smooth muscle. A disproportionate rise in m-AST has been observed in patients with alcoholic liver disease, with ratios of m-AST:total AST up to 4x higher than that seen in patients with viral hepatitis or normal subjects. Abstinence from alcohol results in normalisation of m-AST within two weeks. The mechanism for this is unclear but it may reflect mitochondrial damage by alcohol, as other tests of mitochondrial dysfunction (e.g., α-oxo-isocaproic acid breath test) are also abnormal in alcoholic subjects but not in those with cirrhosis due to other causes. Alternatively, it may be due to interference with clearance of m-AST, since this is also elevated in patients with extrahepatic biliary obstruction.

With progressive liver damage, the pattern of biochemical abnormalities tend to shift to reflect intrahepatic cholestasis and reduced liver function. Plasma ALP becomes moderately elevated (up to 5-fold), bilirubin concentrations rise and hypoalbuminaemia becomes a feature.

OTHER BIOCHEMICAL TESTS

The most promising biochemical marker of alcohol misuse to have appeared in recent years is carbohydrate-deficient transferrin (CDT). Initial observations of the presence of an abnormal form of transferrin (detected by isoelectric focusing) in the cerebrospinal fluid of 80% and plasma of 50% of subjects with alcohol-related cerebellar degeneration have been followed by many studies on the effect of alcohol on transferrin metabolism. It is now known that transferrin exists in the circulation in various forms containing from zero up to nine sialic acid residues. In normal healthy individuals, the trisialo- tetrasialo- and pentasialo- forms predominate, but in subjects misusing alcohol, plasma transferrin often lacks 2-4 of these sialic acid residues. The asialo- and disialo-transferrins are now collectively known as CDT. The mechanism for this altered transferrin microheterogeneity is not entirely clear but may involve decreased activity of glycoprotein glycosyl-transferase and increased activity of sialidase due to a direct effect of alcohol. Suffice it to say that consumption of more than 80 g of alcohol per day for more than seven days consistently causes an elevation of CDT, which then falls to normal over approximately 14 days of abstinence. Initial studies of the value of CDT in clinical practice were hampered by the complexity and semi-quantitative nature of the isoelectric focusing method, but this has now been largely superseded by more practical methods based on micro anion exchange chromatography followed by immunoassay of the separated transferrin fractions. There is still debate about whether CDT measurements should be expressed in absolute terms (mass or units per litre of plasma) or as a percentage of total transferrin. The use of relative measurements avoids false negative or positive results when the total plasma transferrin is below or above the reference range, respectively. Additionally, for absolute measurements there is a difference in the upper reference limits between males (20 U/L) and females (26 U/L), whereas the percentage upper reference limit is the same for both (6%). Many studies have now demonstrated a direct correlation between the plasma CDT concentration and alcohol consumption in males. However, this relationship is much weaker and generally the sensitivity of CDT for detection of alcohol misuse in women is poorer than in men. Whether this relates to changes in transferrin metabolism during the menstrual cycle, possibly hormonal effects on the sialylation process, is not yet clear. The principal value of CDT measurements in clinical practice is for subjects in whom confounding factors (e.g., drug therapy) reduce the specificities of the standard biochemical tests. As CDT appears to be related more to alcohol consumption than to the presence of liver disease, it may have a role in monitoring abstinence in patients.

Other biochemical tests that may be useful include measurement of serotonin metabolites in urine and alterations in plasma lipid profiles. It has been observed that alcohol causes a shift in the metabolism of serotonin from the normal end product 5-hydroxyindoleacetic acid (5-HIAA) to 5-hydroxytryptophol, independently of the presence of liver disease. The ratio of 5-hydroxytryptophol to 5-HIAA in urine collected 12 hours after alcohol consumption has been shown to be increased in a dose dependent manner in both healthy volunteers and known alcohol misusers. Hypertriglyceridaemia is common in heavy drinkers and even moderate alcohol intake increases plasma triglycerides and HDL-cholesterol concentrations, assuming there is no co-existent malnutrition. Plasma cholesterol concentrations are usually normal but may fall as liver damage becomes sufficiently severe to reduce the synthesis of lecithin cholesterol acyltransferase (LCAT). Plasma apolipoprotein A1 (apo-A1) concentrations are elevated in alcoholic steatosis to a greater degree than in patients with established cirrhosis. Apo-A1 has been incorporated into an index with prothrombin time and GGT (the 'PGA index') that can be used to diagnose cirrhosis with a sensitivity and specificity of around 80%.

Additionally, plasma ferritin is often elevated in alcoholic liver disease, either as part of an acute phase response or due to release of the protein from damaged hepatocytes, but the rises are not usually of the magnitude seen in iron overload syndromes. If the ferritin is particularly high (> 500 µg/L), the transferrin saturation and total iron binding capacity (TIBC) should be determined and genotyping performed to exclude underlying hereditary haemochromatosis in either the homozygous or heterozygous states.

IMMUNOLOGICAL TESTS

Hyperglobulinaemia is a common finding in alcohol-induced liver disease. In contrast to other diseases associated with hyperglobulinaemia (Chapter 6), plasma IgA is characteristically disproportionately elevated in about 80% of patients. Plasma IgG may also be moderately raised in those with hepatic parenchymal inflammation but usually to a lesser extent, while IgM concentrations are usually normal or only slightly elevated. Additionally, patients with advanced alcoholic liver disease have a wide range of circulating autoantibodies as well as antibodies reacting with acetaldehyde-protein adducts. The significance of these is poorly understood but the presence of autoantibodies can complicate the differential diagnosis of alcohol-induced liver disease from autoimmune liver diseases (Chapter 6).

HAEMATOLOGICAL TESTS

Mild hypochromic or normochromic anaemia is found in approximately 75% of patients with cirrhosis of any aetiology. Macrocytosis (with or without anaemia) is a relatively insensitive screening test as it occurs in only 20-30% of alcohol misusers in community settings. Also, increased mean cell volume (MCV) can be due to a number of other factors including folate deficiency, recent blood loss and various haemolytic conditions. Increased MCV is more common in female than male alcohol misusers. It is due to the effect of the alcohol on the developing erythroblast and, consequently, may take some months to normalise after abstinence. Leucocytosis occurs in more than 50% of patients with alcoholic hepatitis and leucopenia occurring in about 5%. Thrombocytopenia may occur, either due to impairment of platelet function by alcohol or associated with portal hypertension and hypersplenism in patients with cirrhosis.

Most of the compounds involved in blood clotting are synthezised by the liver. They have turnover times of 1-4 days, in contrast to albumin which has a half-life of about 20 days. Measurement of prothrombin time (INR) is therefore a useful measure of recent changes in hepatic synthetic function. However, the INR is not usually markedly elevated unless there is significant hepatocellular necrosis. Factor V concentrations may be a useful indicator of prognosis as they are often decreased to a greater extent than the prolongation of prothrombin time in patients with severe alcoholic liver disease with a poor outcome.

ENDOCRINOLOGICAL ABNORMALITIES

Men with alcohol-induced cirrhosis have significant sexual dysfunction and are frequently impotent and may have gynaecomastia and testicular atrophy. Although these changes are seen in cirrhosis of all aetiologies, hypogonadism also occurs in alcoholic men without cirrhosis and may be due to direct effects of alcohol on the male reproductive endocrine system. Total plasma testosterone concentration is lower and oestradiol higher in alcoholic cirrhosis than in other types of cirrhosis. Sex hormone binding globulin concentration also is invariably raised. The low plasma testosterone concentration is attributable to a combination of reduced testicular production and increased peripheral conversion to oestradiol. It would be expected that the low circulating testosterone levels should be accompanied by a compensatory increase in pituitary secretion of luteinizing hormone (LH) but this does not always occur, implying that a primary testicular defect is often complicated by hypothalamic-pituitary dysfunction. About 75% of men with cirrhosis have oligospermia and this is (unusually) associated with normal plasma follicle stimulating hormone (FSH) concentrations. Absence of testicular atrophy, a normal LH, or a normal response of LH to luteinizing hormone release hormone (LHRH) predict restoration of sexual function in alcoholic men who abstain from alcohol.

Impaired glucose tolerance is common in patients with cirrhosis of any aetiology, and type 2 diabetes mellitus often develops as the disease progresses. Although the fasting blood glucose is usually normal, the response to a glucose load is within the diabetic range. Chronic pancreatitis leading to development of diabetes is a frequent complication in alcohol misusers whether or not there is hepatic damage. In others, fasting insulin and glucagon concentrations are almost invariably raised, indicating insulin resistance rather than an effect of alcohol on the pancreas. The mechanism appears to be impaired hepatic extraction of insulin and glucose by the liver, together with increased delivery to the systemic circulation as a consequence of porto-systemic circulation. In some cases, profound hypoglycaemia may occur if little or no food is consumed during an alcoholic binge.

Pseudo-Cushing's syndrome is a well recognised endocrinological manifestation of alcoholic liver disease. Patients are typically obese and may have raised plasma cortisol concentrations with loss of the normal diurnal rhythm and increased ACTH secretion. Abstinence will normally correct these abnormalities. Thyroid dysfunction is also common in alcoholic liver disease and many patients have a clinically thyrotoxic appearance with exophthalmia, weight loss and tremor. The rate of thyroxine (T4) secretion is normal but there is depression of 5'-deiodinase activity, which results in a reduction in conversion of T4 to tri-iodothyronine (T3) and an increase in reverse T3 (rT3) production. The circulating concentrations of free T4 and thyrotropin (TSH) are therefore often normal but free T3 is low. The rT3/T3 ratio appears to be a sensitive prognostic indicator in alcoholic liver disease.

PARACETAMOL

Paracetamol (known as acetaminophen in the USA) is currently the most common cause of drug-related hepatic injury in the world. When taken on its own as an analgesic paracetamol appears to be a safe and effective drug with single doses of up to 5g (in adults) not being associated with toxicity. Larger doses, usually taken with parasuicidal intent, are hepatotoxic causing acute hepatic necrosis over the ensuing 36-72 hours. Severe hepatic injury and even death have resulted from paracetamol taken with therapeutic intent in combination with other drugs such as phenytoin, phenobarbitone or other drugs that enhance the cytochrome P-450 system, and in alcoholics in whom the enzyme system may also be induced.

In healthy subjects, more than 90% of an oral dose of paracetamol is eliminated by glucuronidation or sulphation. Less than 5% is metabolized via the cytochrome P-450 pathway (primarily 2EI) to the electrophilic metabolite N-acetyl-p-benzo-quinone imine (NAPQI). NAPQI is rapidly eliminated via conjugation to glutathione (Figure 5.8). In overdose, saturation of the sulphation and glucuronidation pathways results in a greater proportion of paracetamol metabolism being shunted through the oxidative cytochrome P-450 pathway. As glutathione stores become depleted NAPQI remains unconjugated and can interact with hepatic proteins, impairing their function and resulting in cell death.

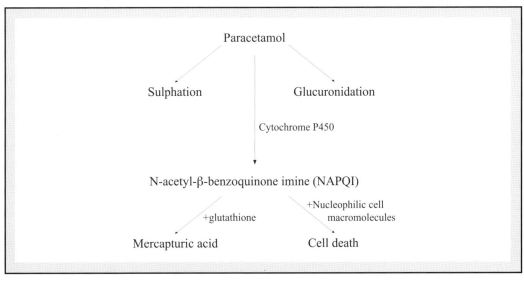

Figure 5.8 Pathway of paracetamol metabolism

The clinical course of paracetamol overdose can be divided into four stages. Within a few hours of ingestion the patient may experience anorexia, nausea and vomiting which can persist for up to 24 hours. Following this patients enter a second stage with remission of symptoms and can remain well for 48 hours. During this phase the plasma aminotransferases rise sharply as hepatic stores of glutathione are depleted and hepatic necrosis occurs. In the third stage plasma bilirubin begins to rise and the prothrombin time becomes prolonged. The patient may then develop encephalopathy rapidly. Acute renal failure, with oliguria or anuria, due to renal tubular necrosis, occurs in 25-30% of untreated patients with significant overdoses. If patients survive they enter the fourth stage with recovery occurring 5-10 days after ingestion. A prognostic scoring system has been derived at King's College Hospital incorporating laboratory and clinical parameters that has a predictive accuracy of 80%. An arterial pH < 7.3 (H^+ concentration > 50 nmol/L), an INR > 6.0, a plasma creatinine > 300 μmol/L and grade III/IV encephalopathy are associated with a poor prognosis for recovery without liver transplantation. An additional prognostic indicator is the molar ratio of factor VIIII to V with a ratio > 30 indicating poor prognosis.

Rapid diagnosis of paracetamol overdose is essential as administration of sulphydryl donor compounds which can substitute for glutathione in the conjugation of NAPQI has been shown to be an effective antidote even as late as 48 hours after ingestion. N-acetylcysteine (Parvolex) is the preferred antidote and can be given either orally or intravenously, although in the latter case hypersensitivity has been reported in up to 10% of recipients. The effective dose of paracetamol taken may be difficult to determine from the history as vomiting may have resulted in some of the ingested drug not being absorbed. The plasma concentration of paracetamol and its clearance rate can be a useful indicator of the likelihood of hepatic damage occurring. Patients with high plasma paracetamol concentrations (> 1 mmol/L at 6 h and > 0.2 mmol/L at 14h after ingestion, 150 and 30 mg/L respectively) will invariably suffer hepatic damage without treatment. Measurements before 4 hours are not helpful as absorption of the drug may be continuing. A guideline for the necessity for treatment based on plasma paracetamol concentrations is shown in Figure 5.9, although some centres will give N-acetylcysteine at lower plasma paracetamol concentrations. Plasma paracetamol concentrations should also be measured in alcoholics presenting with acute hepatitis if their plasma AST is greater than 300 IU/L even if there is no history of paracetamol ingestion.

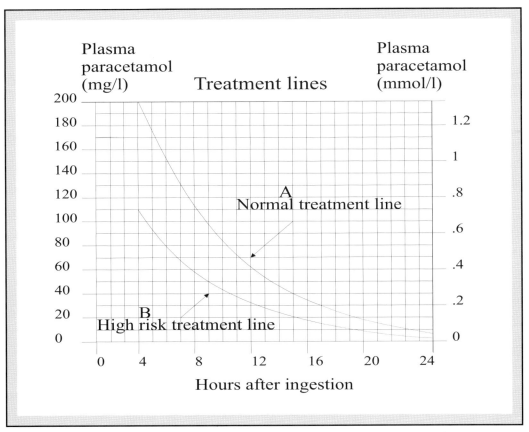

Figure 5.9 **Guidelines for N-acetylcysteine treatment based on plasma paracetamol concentrations**

OTHER DRUGS IMPLICATED IN HEPATOTOXICITY

ANTICONVULSANTS

Among the anticonvulsants, phenytoin (diphenylhydantoin) and valproate (dipropyl-acetic acid) are known to be hepatotoxic. Carbamazepine and felbamate have also been associated with liver damage in some patients. About 20% of patients taking phenytoin show persistent mild elevations of plasma aminotransferases, but a smaller proportion (less than 1%) can develop an acute hepatic illness which may progress to acute hepatic failure. A few fatal cases of phenytoin hepatotoxicity have been reported. There is no relation between the development of hepatic damage and the plasma phenytoin concentration suggesting that hypersensitivity may be the mechanism of injury. Phenytoin is metabolized via the cytochrome P-450 system, which it induces, and it is possible that toxic metabolites could be formed.

In adults sodium valproate appears to be less toxic than phenytoin but 10% of patients show elevated plasma aminotransferases to an extent which is often dose-related. Severe hepatotoxicity with mitochrondrial damage and altered fatty acid oxidation is seen in fewer than 0.01% of patients. A number of fatal cases of valproate hepatotoxicity have been reported, particularly in young patients on polytherapy. Patients typically present with lethargy, anorexia and vomiting and have jaundice, hypoglycaemia and a raised blood ammonia. Such cases are not dose or plasma concentration dependent and may be due to an idiosyncratic reaction to the drug. The aminotransferases are not markedly raised. Histological features include microvesicular steatosis with centrilobular necrosis.

Carbamazepine has been reported to cause elevations in plasma aminotransferases in up to 20% of patients, 6-8 weeks after commencing therapy. Carbamazepine is also metabolized via the cytochrome P-450 system and it is possible the metabolite, 10,11-epoxide, is involved in hepatic injury. Felbamate has been associated with severe liver damage in a few cases but more data is required before it can be conclusively labelled as hepatotoxic.

ANTI-INFLAMMATORY DRUGS
Paracetamol hepatotoxicity has already been discussed. Salicylate (aspirin) taken in normal therapeutic doses is seldom hepatotoxic but a mild asymptomatic, reversible hepatotoxicity which is dose dependent has been reported. Damage is predominantly hepatocellular, with raised plasma aminotransferases and normal or only mildly elevated plasma bilirubin and ALP. Among reported cases of salicylate hepatotoxicity 66% have plasma salicylate concentrations > 250 mg/L (1.8 mmol/L) and 90% > 150 mg/L (1.1 mmol/L). Overdoses rarely cause hepatic injury, whilst rheumatoid arthritis patients seem most prone, suggesting damage may be due to a cumulative effect. Salicylate has also been implicated in the development of a Reye-like syndrome in children.

The majority of the non-steroidal anti-inflammatory drugs (NSAIDs) appear to be relatively free from hepatotoxicity, particularly in view of the widespread availability of these agents. Although elevations in plasma aminotransferases have been reported in a varying proportion of patients taking NSAIDs these were typically in patients with rheumatoid arthritis or systemic lupus erythematosus (SLE), conditions in which elevated liver enzymes are frequently seen in untreated patients. Diclofenac has been shown to elevate plasma aminotransferases in some patients with osteoarthritis (80% female). Histologically the liver damage is predominantly acute peripheral or centrilobular necrosis and probably reflects an idiosyncratic mechanism. It is recommended that plasma aminotransferases be measured at 2-3 month intervals in such patients. Sulindac can cause a mixed pattern of hepatocellular damage and cholestasis in the first 6-8 weeks after commencing therapy. The majority of cases of sulindac hepatotoxicity have been women; it is likely that the mechanism is hypersensitivity. Co-existent pancreatitis has been reported. Very few cases of hepatic injury, considering their widespread use, have been seen with ibuprofen, flurbiprofen, naproxen or the oxicam (enolic acids) family of drugs.

ANTIMICROBIAL AGENTS

ANTIBIOTICS

The hepatotoxic potential of the tetracyclines is well known but is really only of academic interest now as these drugs are used relatively infrequently in current practice. Erythromycin may occasionally cause hepatic damage. The laboratory picture is that of cholestatic hepatitis with only moderate (< 10-fold) elevations of plasma aminotransferases, often associated with an eosinophilia. The latter, together with an urticarial rash which is a common presenting symptom, suggests that toxicity is related to hypersensitivity. Augmentin® (amoxicillin clavulanic acid) is known to be hepatotoxic in some patients, resulting in a cholestatic picture. Interestingly this has only been reported in adults, usually after 4-6 weeks of therapy and probably reflects hypersensitivity. The severe hypersensitivity reactions commonly seen with penicillin itself are only rarely associated with hepatic damage but other penicillins, such as carbenicillin, oxacillin and phenoxymethylpenicillin, reportedly cause parenchymal liver injury (with or without cholestasis) occasionally when given intravenously in large doses. Co-trimoxazole (Septrin®) often causes mild elevations in ALP and GGT, but instances of hyperbilirubinaemia or severe liver damage seem to be very rare.

ANTI-FUNGAL AGENTS

Ketaconazole, and less frequently itraconazole, have been reported to have mild, asymptomatic, to severe hepatoxicity with acute or hyperacute liver failure, although this appears rare (1 in 15,000 patients). Damage is predominantly hepatocellular, with or without cholestasis, and among reported cases there is a 2:1 female to male ratio with most patients being over 40 years of age.

ANTI-PARASITIC AGENTS

Hepatotoxicity among the anti-parasitic agents is relatively rare but the organic antimonials and chlorinated hydrocarbons, used as antihelminthics, have long been known to cause liver damage. The antischistosomal drugs hycanthone and niridazole have been reported to produce hepatocellular necrosis as has piper-azine.

ANTI TUBERCULOUS DRUGS

First-line treatment of tuberculosis usually involves rifampicin and isoniazid or both, together with other drugs. When taken separately, up to 4% of patients receiving rifampicin and about 1% of those taking isoniazid develop some degree of hepatocellular damage. Rifampicin competes with bilirubin for transport across the liver cell and conjugated or unconjugated hyperblilirubinaemia can often occur as the sole biochemical abnormality but, in cases of severe hepatotoxicty, will normally be accompanied by high plasma aminotransferase activities.

ANTI RETROVIRAL AGENTS

Most of the drugs used against HIV infections have not been in use for long enough for reliable data on hepatotoxicity to have become available. Zidovudine has been associated with some hepatic-like events and with decompensation of pre-existing chronic hepatitis in some patients, and with hepatomegaly and steatosis in others. It is, however, difficult in most AIDS patients to determine whether hepatotxicity is due to an individual drug or to multidrug interactions and/or underlying systemic disease. Although didanosine caused elevations in plasma aminotransferases and several cases of acute hepatic failure in early clinical trials, these occurred in the high-dose arm and the prevalence of other side-effects resulted in lower dosage regimens being introduced into clinical practice. There are, as yet, insufficient data to establish whether zalcitabine (ddc) or stavudine (d4T) exhibit any hepatotoxicity.

CARDIOVASCULAR DRUGS

Among the various different classes of drugs in this category there are several for which hepatotoxicity has been well documented (methyldopa, amiodarone) and others where only rare instances of hepatic damage have been recorded angiotensin converting enzyme (ACE) inhibitors, quinidine, procainamide. Methyldopa hepatotoxicity is a well recognised entity, ranging from asymptomatic increases in plasma aminotransferases to active hepatitis and even fatal necrosis. Approximately 5% of patients on methyldopa have a raised plasma AST but only 1% progress to actual liver disease, which in 80% of cases is an acute hepatocellular condition, in 5% cholestatic and in 15% has the characteristics of chronic hepatitis. In those cases with chronic damage, presentation is often virtually indistinguishable from that of autoimmune hepatitis with LE cell phenomena, hyperglobulinaemia, non-organ-specific autoantibodies and anti-LSP antibodies. Among the β-blockers, labetalol has been linked to hepatotoxicity and it is recommended that it is not used in patients with pre-existing liver disease.

Amiodarone is known to be hepatotoxic with transient elevations in the plasma aminotransferases occurring in up to 40% of patients. In a small proportion, hepatomegaly occurs and may progress to cirrhosis. In about 1% of patients, liver damage presenting as pseudoalcoholic hepatitis occurs. Current recommendations are that the plasma aminotransferases should be measured prior to treatment and at regular intervals thereafter, and that the drug should be withdrawn if rises to more than twice the upper reference limit occur. Acute hepatic injury has been observed following intravenous loading with amiodarone. It is not clear, however, whether this is directly related to amiodarone or is an allergic reaction to the organic surfactant used in the carrier medium.

Hepatotoxicity is the most common of the serious side effects associated with use of the HMG-CoA inhibitors (statins). Asymptomatic elevations of plasma aminotransferases occurs in 1-2% of patients within 12-18 months of initiating therapy. These usually resolve on discontinuing the drug and a direct dose relationship has been shown for lovastatin. There is no evidence of hepatotoxicity for the current generation of fibrates and only rare reports for nicotinic acid.

ANAESTHETIC AGENTS

Liver damage associated with halothane anaesthesia has been recognised since the 1960s. The exact frequency of hepatitis caused by halothane is unknown, but severe hepatic damage reportedly occurs in about 1 in 35,000 anaesthetics and in about 1 in 3,700 patients following multiple exposures. Less severe clinical hepatitis probably occurs more often and minor (2-4 fold) elevations in plasma aminotransferases are common. The severe reaction to halothane is idiosyncratic. Anti-LSP antibodies are found at high titre in about half of the patients during the acute phase. More specifically, a plasma antibody that reacts with a rabbit liver antigen altered in vivo by halothane can be detected in most cases. Of the newer flurane anaesthetics, hepatitis has been reported with enflurane but only at a low incidence of 1 in 800,000 exposures. It is not clear yet whether sevoflurane or isoflurane are hepatotoxic.

IMMUNOSUPPRESSIVE DRUGS

The hepatotoxicity of methotrexate, widely used in the treatment of severe psoriasis, is well recognised and seems to be exacerbated by concomitant alcohol consumption or complicating factors such as diabetes or renal impairment. High dose acute methotrexate therapy causes a reversible increase in plasma AST activity but does not lead to chronic liver disease, whereas daily oral methotrexate induces hepatic steatosis and fibrosis that can progress to cirrhosis. Hepatotoxicity appears, therefore, to be a function of the cumulative dose of methotrexate. Current recommended practice has been to undertake a liver biopsy after every 1.5g cumulative dose of methotrexate or if the basic liver biochemistry tests become markedly abnormal. Measurement of the plasma procollagen-III peptide

N-terminal (PIIINP) may permit a reduction in the number of liver biopsies carried out to monitor methotrexate therapy. An increase in plasma PIIINP has been shown to be related to increasing hepatic fibrosis and would be an indicator for a confirmatory liver biopsy. In a patient with normal liver biochemistry tests and a stable PIIINP concentration, biopsy can be delayed.

Hepatotoxicity associated with use of cyclosporin A (CyA) has been seen after renal, cardiac and bone transplantation. In liver transplant recipients it is difficult to determine if liver abnormalities are related to CyA use or rejection. Biliary calculi are found in a higher proportion of patients on CyA than on other drugs. It has been suggested that CyA causes the formation of 'biliary sludge' which leads to cholestasis. There appears to be a degree of dose relationship as cholestatic liver disease is more common where the blood CyA concentration is kept in the range 200-400 µg/L than below 200 µg/L. Tacrolimus does not appear to be hepatotoxic.

Azathioprine is known to have some degree of hepatotoxicity causing cholestasis with or without necrosis. A particular histological feature is nodular regenerative hyperplasia. Portal hypertension may be a late affect of azathioprine hepatotoxicity, occurring in possibly up to 10% of patients following liver transplantation.

PSYCHOTROPIC DRUGS

Psychotropic drugs are well-known hepatotoxins. The phenothiazines, benzodiazepines and tricyclic anti-depressants tend to be cholestatic agents, while monoamine oxidase inhibitors are more likely to produce hepatocellular damage. Chlorpromazine jaundice is a particularly well-recognised complication and up to 2% of patients taking this drug are likely to develop the syndrome 1-4 weeks after commencing treatment. There is a pronounced hypercholesterolaemia and continued use can lead to a cirrhosis which resembles primary biliary cirrhosis and only resolves slowly on stopping the drug. It has been postulated that the mechanism is via drug-induced impairment of bile flow. Among the butyrophenones a hypersensitivity-induced cholestatic liver injury can be found in approximately 0.2% of patients taking haloperidol.

Benzodiazepines rarely cause a cholestatic hepatitis, sometimes accompanied by eosinophilia. Hypersensitivity-related cholestasis can be seen in 0.5-1.0% of patients taking tricyclic antidepressants. There are only a few anecdotal reports of elevated plasma aminotransferases with the serotonin reuptake inhibitor class of compounds (SSRIs)

OCCUPATIONAL, ENVIRONMENTAL AND OTHER AGENTS

The list of potential hepatotoxins with which we come into contact in our daily lives is far too long to reproduce here and only a few examples are given to illustrate the range of these compounds.

Industrial chemicals are an obvious source of potential hepatotoxins. This category includes trichloroethylene (Trilene®) which is used as a solvent in adhesives and which has been known to cause hepatocellular damage in young people indulging in 'glue-sniffing'. Although now rare, accidental poisoning with carbon tetrachloride may still be encountered. Some pesticides, and compounds used in the paint and plastics industries cause hepatic injury in various ways.

In the plant world, there are numerous compounds that are hepatotoxic in man. These range from the Senecio and Heliotropium alkaloids (which cause veno-occlusive disease) to the mushroom toxins (of which that produced by the 'black-cap' mushroom, Amanita phalloides, is perhaps the most frequent cause of mushroom poisoning) and to the aflatoxin family of compounds. The latter are produced by fungi that grow on groundnuts stored in damp conditions. They are potent carcinogens and, at higher doses, can be directly hepatotoxic.

FURTHER READING

Alcoholic liver disease. Balliere's Clinical Gastroenterology Vol 7 No. 3 (PC Hayes Ed) 1993.

Conigrave KM, Saunders JB, Whitfield JB. Diagnostic tests for alcoholic consumption. Alcohol Alcoholism 1995; **30:** 13-26.

Drug-induced liver disease. Gastro Clinics North America 1995; **24:** 730-800

Eadie MY, McKinnon GE, Dunston PR, MacLanghlin D, Dickinson RG.Valproate metabolism during hepatotoxicity associated with the drug. Quart J Med 1990; **284:** 1229-40.

Harrison PM, Keays R, Bray GP, Alexander GJM, Williams R. Improved outcome of paracetamol-induced fulminant hepatic failure by late administration of acetylcysteine. Lancet 1990; **335:** 1572-3.

Larrey D, Pageaux GP. Genetic predisposition to drug-induced hepatotoxicity. J. Hepatol 1997; **26(Suppl 2):** 12-21.

Ray DC, Drummond GB. Halothane hepatitis. Br J Anaesth 1991; **67:** 84-9.

Stibler H. Carbohydrate-deficient transferrin in serum: a new marker potentially harmful alcohol consumption reviewed. Clin Chem 1991; **37:** 2029-37.

Van Pelt FNAM, Straub P, Manns MP. Molecular basis of drug-induced immunological liver injury. Sem Liver Dis 1995; **15:** 283-300.

Zimmerman HJ. Hepatotoxicity: The adverse effects of drugs and other chemicals on the liver. New York Appleton-Century Crofts 1978.

Chapter 6

Autoimmune liver disease

INTRODUCTION

Three chronic liver disorders are usually classified under the heading of autoimmune liver disease: autoimmune hepatitis (AIH), primary biliary cirrhosis (PBC) and primary sclerosing cholangitis (PSC). These conditions were considered to be quite rare but, with increasing awareness and advances in diagnostic techniques, they are being diagnosed more frequently and have been reported in all major ethnic groups. Data on their incidence and prevalence worldwide are lacking but in Europe the combined prevalence is probably about 250 cases per million of the population.

AIH is a disease affecting the hepatic parenchyma. PBC and PSC primarily affect the bile ducts, although some parenchymal liver damage may be seen at certain stages in both. In PBC, it is the small interlobular bile ducts inside the liver that are damaged, whereas in PSC either or both the extrahepatic and intrahepatic ducts may be affected - leading to a characteristic pattern of strictures and beading of the ducts that can be visualised by cholangiography. All three are progressive disorders that eventually lead to cirrhosis in most cases. In contrast to cirrhosis due to other causes, development of hepatocellular carcinoma (HCC) in AIH is very rare. HCC is more common (but still comparatively rare) in PBC and PSC but, in PSC, there is a high risk of cholangiocarcinoma (Chapter 7).

Most of the signs and symptoms of these diseases are non-specific. Lethargy (often profound) is a prominent feature and this should be borne in mind in the differential diagnosis of chronic fatigue syndromes. It may be accompanied by epigastric pain, fever and chills, arthralgia, myalgia and/or jaundice. Pruritus (itching) is sometimes a feature in AIH and PSC but is a particularly common presenting symptom of PBC. The pathogenesis of pruritus in PBC and other cholestatic diseases is unknown but recent evidence suggests that it can be relieved by opioid antagonists and may be mediated through the central nervous system. Osteodystrophy is a late manifestation of both PBC and PSC. However, within each disorder, there is wide variation between patients in the severity and rate of progression of disease and it is now recognised that they can all have quite prolonged asymptomatic (or pre-symptomatic) phases. These asymptomatic cases usually come to light through routine health screening or during investigation of some other condition and there is now evidence that, in a minority of patients, the liver disease may never become clinically significant. Conversely, AIH can present as a severe acute hepatitis that can be difficult to distinguish clinically from acute viral hepatitis, while some cases of PSC present with features of acute cholangitis. However, acute presentation of PBC has not been reported.

An important distinction between the three conditions is seen in their responses to immunosuppressive drug therapy. The great majority of patients with AIH show a striking response to treatment with corticosteroids with or without azathioprine (or occasionally other agents) and can be maintained in remission for long periods on low doses of these drugs. This does not represent a 'cure' because most patients relapse sooner or later when treatment is stopped and many will require some form of therapy for life. Nonetheless, recent studies have shown that, for carefully managed AIH patients, life expectancy is probably not significantly different from that in an age- and sex-matched normal population. In contrast, numerous clinical trials of a wide range of immunosuppressive agents over many years have failed to show any marked benefit of immunosuppressive therapy in PBC or PSC, other than occasionally in patients with features that overlap with those of AIH (see 'Overlapping Disorders', below), and both of these diseases progress inexorably in many cases to a point where liver transplantation becomes the only therapeutic option.

Evidence of autoimmunity in these conditions includes hypergammaglobulinaemia and high titres of circulating autoantibodies, but elevations in Plasma immunoglobulins and autoantibodies (albeit usually at lower titres) are also frequently seen in patients with acute or chronic viral hepatitis (Chapter 3), in alcoholic liver disease (Chapter 5) and in some metabolic liver disorders (Chapter 4). Additionally, there is a wide range of drugs that can produce idiosyncratic reactions with manifestations of autoimmune liver disease (Chapter 5). Diagnosis of AIH, PBC and PSC therefore requires careful exclusion of these other conditions, together with biochemical liver tests and screening for autoantibodies. Testing for immunogenetic markers (HLA phenotypes) is not usually routinely undertaken but can be useful for reinforcing the diagnosis. However, definitive diagnoses can only be made by histological examination of liver biopsy specimens and cholangiography is often required for the differential diagnosis of PSC, especially in children.

AUTOIMMUNE HEPATITIS

AIH is a disorder that predominantly affects females (F:M ratio 4:1). It fulfils most of the criteria for a classic organ-specific autoimmune disease. In addition to the presenting signs and symptoms discussed above, there is often evidence of endocrinopathy including dysmenorrhoea in females, hirsutism and acneiform rashes. Up to 30% of patients have a concomitant autoimmune disorder, most frequently thyroid disease (Hashimoto's thyroiditis or Graves' disease) or rheumatoid arthritis. There is also often a family history of these or other autoimmune conditions, although familial AIH is very rare. Early studies noted its association with circulating lupus erythematosus (LE) cells (phagocytic leukocytes containing large, Feulgen-positive, cytoplasmic inclusions comprising cell nuclei with adherent 7S-IgG and complement components that have been extruded from damaged lymphocytes and engulfed by the phagocytes) and for many years it was termed 'lupoid' hepatitis. However, it is now known that LE cells occur in only a relatively small proportion of AIH patients and that the disease is distinct from systemic lupus erythematosus (SLE).

AIH can develop at any age but the large majority of patients present above the age of 40 years. In children and young adults it tends to be more severe and more difficult to control with immunosuppressive therapy, and to progress more rapidly to cirrhosis, than in older subjects. Nonetheless, about 30% of patients in all age groups already have established cirrhosis when they first present, which is in keeping with the observation that the disease often has a prolonged pre-symptomatic phase. Current recommendations are that patients should be classified as having 'definite' or 'probable' AIH according to how closely the presenting features correspond to those of classic ('lupoid') AIH.

BIOCHEMICAL LIVER TESTS
In AIH, the plasma biochemical liver tests typically show a 'hepatitic' pattern, with raised aminotransferase activities and bilirubin concentrations but normal or only mildly elevated alkaline phosphatase (ALP). Gammaglutamyl transferase (GGT) activities may also be elevated (occasionally quite markedly) but are of uncertain clinical significance. However, even in patients with severe disease, the aminotransferase activities can vary widely - from 2 to 50 times the upper reference limits. Furthermore, AIH is typically a fluctuating condition in which the signs, symptoms and plasma biochemical abnormalities wax and wane with a periodicity of anything from a few months to one or two years, despite ongoing necroinflammation of the liver. Therefore, a low aminotransferase activity does not necessarily indicate mild or inactive disease.

Plasma albumin concentration is usually normal but globulin concentrations are characteristically elevated. The hyperglobulinaemia in AIH is due mainly to a marked and selective elevation of plasma IgG concentration and this is one of the diagnostic criteria for the condition. Plasma IgA and IgM concentrations are usually normal, although IgM may be moderately elevated in severe disease (Figure 6.1).

Laboratory findings in autoimmune liver disease			
Serum parameter	AIH	PBC	PSC
Aminotransferases (AST or ALT)	+ or +++	N or +	N or +
Bilirubin	N or ++	++ or +++	+ or ++
Alkaline phosphatase	N or +	+++	+ or ++
Gammaglutamyltransferase	N or ++	+ or ++	+ or ++
Immunoglobulins:			
IgG	++ or +++	N or +	+ or ++
IgM	N or +	++ or +++	N or +
IgA	N or +	N or +	N or +
Autoantibodies (% with titres > 1:40):			
ANA or SMA	80%	30-40%	20%
LKM1	3-4%	0	0
AMA	0	>90%	0
N = normal, + = mildly, ++ = moderately, +++ = markedly elevated			

Figure 6.1 Typical laboratory findings at presentation in patients with autoimmune hepatitis (AIH), primary biliary cirrhosis (PBC) and primary sclerosing cholangitis (PSC)

AUTOANTIBODIES

About 80% of patients with AIH present with significant titres (> 1:40) of antinuclear (ANA) and/or smooth muscle (SMA) autoantibodies. These are not specific to AIH but they form part of the diagnostic criteria. Up to 90% also reportedly have perinuclear staining anti-neutrophil cytoplasmic antibodies (pANCA) which, again, are not specific to AIH. A small sub-group (3-4%) of patients have so-called type 1 antiliver-kidney microsomal antibodies (anti-LKM1), usually without ANA and SMA. Titres of ANA and SMA often fall, and the antibodies may disappear, with response to immunosuppressive therapy but anti-LKM1 usually persists at high titre. In addition to these 'conventional' autoantibodies, so-called because they are routinely determined by most clinical immunology laboratories, patients with autoimmune liver disease have a wide range of autoantibodies reacting with various liver-derived antigens. Patients with anti-mitochondrial autoantibodies (AMA) should not be considered to have AIH (see 'Overlapping syndromes').

It has become the convention to designate anti-LKM1 positive cases as 'Type 2' AIH to distinguish them from the ANA/SMA-positive ('Type 1' AIH) patients. Type 2 patients are usually young females with severe disease. However, the clinical utility of this classification is uncertain because it is not exclusive - the great majority of young females with severe AIH are in fact Type 1 - and long-term outcome is similar in both types. Other subdivisions of AIH based on autoantibody profiles have been proposed but have not been widely adopted.

ANTI-NUCLEAR ANTIBODIES (ANA)

Anti-nuclear antibodies comprise a wide spectrum of autoantibodies that react with various antigens associated with cell nuclei. Screening for ANAs is usually performed by indirect immunofluorescence on frozen sections of rodent tissues or on other appropriate substrates such as HEp2 cells or the protozoan *Crithidia luciliae* (which has a modified mitochondrion, the kinetoplast, thought to contain only double-stranded DNA). Techniques for ANA screening differ between laboratories and clinical interpretation of results depends on a knowledge of which method has been used. Titres of ANA > 1:40 are considered significant in adults with liver disease when rodent tissues are used as substrates but with the more sensitive method of detection using HEp2 cells titres < 1:80 are not usually regarded as significant.

Depending on the substrate employed, four main patterns of immunofluorescent staining are recognised:

- homogeneous, diffuse staining over the whole nucleus;
- speckled, a particulate pattern which may be fine and uniform, granular and clumpy, or dots;
- peripheral, outlining the rim of the nucleus;
- nucleolar.

The pattern of staining can provide a clue to the target antigen involved as well as to the disease. Thus, the homogeneous pattern is typical of that given by ANAs in the sera of patients with systemic lupus erythematosus (SLE) that react with DNA, histone proteins, or chromatin - although these are not specific to SLE. The uniform speckled pattern is characteristic of the anti-centromere antibody associated with progressive systemic sclerosis (PSS) and, more particularly, with the CREST syndrome (calcinosis, Raynaud's phenomenon, oesophageal dysmotility, sclerodactyly and telangiectasia), while the clumpy speckled pattern is seen with (but is not exclusive to) antibodies against the ribonucleoproteins Ro and La in SLE, Sjögren's syndrome and mixed connective tissue disorders. The peripheral pattern is given by antibodies that react with nuclear membrane components (particularly the lamins) in various disorders, while nucleolar staining is seen with ANAs in PSS. Some specialist laboratories will provide an 'ANA profile', using additional techniques including enzyme-linked immunoassays (ELISAs), radioimmunoassays (RIAs) and immunoblotting to detail the antigenic specificities of the ANAs detected by routine immunofluorescence. ANAs in AIH commonly show homogeneous staining but all of the other patterns are also frequently seen. However, the different patterns of staining and antigenic specificities appear to have no clinical significance in AIH.

ANTI-SMOOTH MUSCLE ANTIBODIES (SMA)
Smooth muscle antibodies (SMA) react with a variety of cytoskeletal components (CSCs) including F-actin, desmin, myosin, tubulin and vimentin. In most clinical immunology laboratories, SMA is routinely detected by indirect immunofluorescence on composite frozen sections of rat stomach, kidney and liver, on which the antibodies stain the gastric muscularis mucosa, the renal blood vessels as well as (to a lesser extent) the glomeruli and tubular epithelial cells, and microfilaments in liver cells. Because many CSCs are insoluble, liquid-phase assays such as immunodiffusion, immunoblotting, ELISAs or RIAs cannot be used to define the full range of specificities of different SMAs. To achieve this, some laboratories employ immunofluorescence on cryostat sections of liver from rats chronically injected with phalloidin, or primary cultures of various cell lines that have been treated with drugs such as colchicine and vinblastine, to enhance expression of various CSCs.

SMAs of all three immunoglobulin classes and various specificities are found in sera from patients with a wide range of hepatic and non-hepatic disorders. High titre anti-actin antibodies of the IgG isotype are particularly frequent in AIH and are considered by some authorities to define Type 1 disease. These anti-actin antibodies react with F-actin and this is a major distinction from alcoholic liver disease (Chapter 5) in which low titre SMA are found that react predominantly with G-actin. However, anti-F-actin occurs quite frequently in other diseases. Furthermore, anti-F-actin positive cases account for only about 50% of patients who otherwise qualify for a diagnosis of Type 1 AIH. Thus reliance on anti-actin specificity can lead to missed diagnoses of AIH.

PERINUCLEAR ANTI-NEUTROPHIL CYTOPLASMIC ANTIBODIES (pANCA)

Anti-neutrophil cytoplasmic antibodies (ANCA) are a family of antibodies that react with a range of antigens in neutrophils and monocytes. When ethanol-fixed neutrophils are used as the substrate, the patterns of staining of the nuclei by indirect immunofluorescence can be classified into two distinct types: i) cytoplasmic (cANCA) and ii) peripheral (pANCA). Experience is necessary to distinguish the cANCA pattern from staining due to other autoantibodies such as AMA, but the distinction can usually be made on the basis that other autoanti-bodies also stain cells other than neutrophils and monocytes. The perinuclear staining by pANCA can also be seen with some antinuclear antibodies but can be distinguished from these by repeating the test on formaldehyde-fixed cells, on which pANCA give cytoplasmic staining. cANCA was first described in Wegener's granulomatosis and is now known to react mainly with the neutral serine protease proteinase 3. By far the most common of the classic pANCAs are those that react with myeloperoxidase but several other antigens are also recog-nised, including (glucuronidase, cathepsin G, elastase, lactoferrin and lysozyme. Several atypical ANCAs have been described, some of which react with nuclear lamins and with the lamin B receptor, but their clinical significance has not yet been elucidated.

LIVER-KIDNEY MICROSOMAL ANTIBODIES (ANTI-LKM)

Four autoantibodies, designated anti-LKM1 to anti-LKM4, that react with micro-somal antigens in liver and kidney have been described in different diseases (Figure 6.2). The LKM antibodies give a fine granular staining of the cytoplasm of hepatocytes and a slightly more irregular pattern on kidney that can be confused with staining due to AMA. The different anti-LKMs give subtly different staining patterns that require an experienced eye to distinguish from each other and from the staining given by AMA. However, the distinction from AMA by routine immunofluorescence can usually be made by testing on sections of other tissues, such as stomach, which are stained by AMA but not by the anti-LKMs.

The target antigens of these four LKM antibodies have now been identified. Anti-LKM1, which reacts with the cytochrome P450 isoenzyme 2D6, is most particu-larly associated with the 3-4% of patients with so-called Type 2 AIH. Similar autoantibodies can be found in 36% of patients with chronic hepatitis C virus (HCV) infection but appear to react with different epitopes (see 'Overlapping Syndromes'). Anti-LKM2 is directed at a different cytochrome isoform, P450 2C9, and occurs in patients with tienilic acid induced hepatitis. Anti-LKM3, which reacts with members of the family of UDP-glucuronosyl transferases, occurs in about 15% of patients with chronic infection with the hepatitis D (delta) virus but can also be found together with anti-LKM1 in about 10% of Type 2 AIH patients. Anti-LKM4 reacts with cytochrome P450 2A6 and is found in patients with a rare genetically determined disease, autoimmune polyglandular syndrome type 1 (APS-1), which presents in early childhood and is associated with features of AIH in 10-20% of cases. This antibody appears to be an indicator of liver involvement in APS-1. None of these antibodies is known to occur in diseases other than the above.

Liver-kidney microsomal antibodies (anti-LKMs)		
Antibody	**Target antigen**	**Disease association**
Anti-LKM1	Cytochrome P450 2D6	'Type 2' AIH
Anti-LKM2	Cytochrome P450 2C9	Tienilic acid induced hepatitis
Anti-LKM3	UDP-glucuronosyl transferases	Chronic hepatitis D
Anti-LKM4	Cytochrome P450 2A6	Autoimmune polyglandular syndrome type 1

Figure 6.2 Antigenic specificities and disease associations of liver-kidney microsomal antibodies (anti-LKMs)

AUTOANTIBODIES AGAINST LIVER ANTIGENS

Two of the earliest autoantibodies to be described that react with liver-derived antigens were an antibody (liver membrane antibody, LMA) that gave a smooth linear immunofluorescent staining of the surfaces of isolated hepatocytes and another (anti-LSP) that reacted with a crude preparation of liver membrane fragments known as 'liver-specific membrane lipoprotein' (LSP). However, both are now only of historic interest. In recent years several other autoantibodies have been identified which appear to be more specific to liver disease, and to AIH in particular, than ANA, SMA or pANCA. Of greatest current interest are antibodies reacting with: i) a liver cytosolic antigen (LC1); ii) a 'soluble liver antigen' (SLA); and iii) the hepatic asialo-glyco-protein receptor (ASGP-R). LC1 is a 60 kDa liver-specific component which appears to be predominantly located in periportal hepatocytes and which has very recently been identified as formiminotransferase cyclodeaminase. SLA is not liver-specific but is found at highest concentration in liver and was reported to be glutathione-S-transferases, although this has been disputed. The ASGP-R is a receptor which is involved in binding and endocytosis of galactose-terminating asialoglycoproteins. It has been shown to be the major liver-specific component of the LSP preparation and to be an important target of both humoral and cellular (CD4+ T cell) immune reactions in AIH. It seems to be preferentially expressed at high density on the surfaces of periportal hepatocytes in vivo and, if it is indeed a major target of tissue-damaging autoreactions, this pattern of distribution may account for the characteristic periportal liver injury seen in AIH.

Anti-ASGP-R occurs at high titres in almost all AIH patients who have active disease but is also found at similar titres in patients with other liver disorders who have active periportal necroinflammation (interface hepatitis). Thus anti-ASGP-R appears to be more a marker of this histological feature than of AIH per se. Anti-SLA and anti-LC1 are found less frequently (20-50% of patients) but seem to be more specific for AIH, although anti-LC1 also occurs in some patients with chronic hepatitis C. Tests for these three autoantibodies are not yet commercially available but it is likely that they will constitute a new generation of diagnostic markers of AIH when techniques for their detection can be developed for routine application. They have the advantages over the 'conventional' autoantibodies that, in addition to being more specifically related to liver disease, titres correlate much more closely with histologically assessed disease activity (independently of plasma aminotransferase activities) and they are therefore useful for monitoring responses to immunosuppressive therapy. Importantly also, they are found in many of the approximately 20% of AIH patients who present without ANA, SMA or anti-LKM1 antibodies.

HISTOLOGY

The characteristic histological picture in AIH is that of a periportal (interface) hepatitis, with a dense inflammatory infiltrate in the portal tracts, composed mainly of lymphocytes (predominantly CD4+) and plasma cells, spilling out into the surrounding parenchyma with what is described as 'piecemeal necrosis' of the periportal hepatocytes. Similar lesions can be seen in other liver diseases, including acute and chronic viral hepatitis. However, in AIH, morphological features (such as bile duct damage, or granulomas) which are more usually associated with other liver disorders are absent. Depending on the severity and duration of the necroinflammation, varying degrees of fibrosis or established cirrhosis are often evident. Regenerating nodules and bile ductule proliferation are also frequently seen (even in the early stages in severe disease) but are not specific to AIH.

IMMUNOGENETIC MARKERS

There is substantial evidence that genetic factors are involved in susceptibility to AIH. In northern European caucasoids, the disease is strongly linked with inheritance of the A1-B8-DR3 haplotype and particularly with the DR3 and DR4 allotypes, which are also found in association with other autoimmune diseases. Other HLA associations with AIH have been noted in other ethnic populations but have yet to be confirmed. It has also been reported that, in DR3-positive AIH patients with anti-LKM1 antibodies, there is a significantly increased frequency of HLA B14 and of the silent complement gene C4A-Q0 at the C4A locus. However, possession of C4A-Q0 is not confined to this group. It also occurs in patients with Type 1 AIH and, in common with a number of other autoimmune diseases, is associated with an isolated partial deficiency of the C4 complement component which is often inherited in linkage with HLA A1-B8-DR3. Additionally, a highly significant association between AIH and polymorphisms in the genes of two pro-inflammatory cytokines (TNF-α and IL-RA) has very recently been described, suggesting that genetic control of cytokine production may be a factor in AIH.

The DR3 allotype occurs more frequently in younger AIH patients with severe disease while DR4 is mostly associated with an older age at onset and with generally milder disease that is easier to control with immunosuppressive drug therapy. In Japan, where DR3 is very rare in the normal population, the primary HLA association is with DR4 and almost all patients are in the older age groups, with a peak onset at 50-60 years of age. DR3 and DR4 are seldom inherited together as a haplotype in AIH and this apparent segregation of these two allotypes with age at presentation and severity of disease suggests that there may be two genetically distinct populations of patients with AIH. HLA typing is not a routine part of the diagnostic work-up in liver disease but, since almost all northern European caucasoid and Japanese AIH patients have either DR3 or DR4, the presence of these markers can add weight to the diagnosis (especially in ANA/SMA/anti-LKM1 negative patients) and they may also be of value prognostically.

PRIMARY BILIARY CIRRHOSIS

PBC is predominantly a disease of post-menopausal women. Ninety-five percent of patients are female and the median age at presentation is 55 years. It is a slowly progressive disease which is undoubtedly associated with gross immunological abnormalities, but whether it is truly an autoimmune condition is still uncertain. In addition to hypergammaglobulinaemia and circulating autoantibodies, the disorder is associated with circulating immune complexes and chronic activation of complement; patients are generally anergic to parenteral challenge with exogenous antigens; they have defects in suppressing plasma IgM production and in switching from a primary (IgM) to a secondary (IgG) immune response, and they have circulating T lymphocytes that recognise normal biliary tract antigens in vitro. As in AIH, there is quite often a history of other autoimmune conditions, particularly thyroid disease and rheumatological disorders, in the patients and/or their first-degree relatives. On the other hand, as noted above, no satisfactory response to immunosuppressive therapy has been demonstrated in the great majority of PBC patients. Also in contrast to AIH, there is no clear association with inheritance of the 'autoimmune' HLA haplotype (A1-B8-DR3) or the DR3 or DR4 allotypes and the most consistent finding has been an association with DR8. The possibility that PBC is a consequence of an abnormal immune response to an infection is suggested by the well recognised geographical clustering of cases, with the occasional occurrence of the disease in mothers and daughters, and an increased incidence in immigrants from areas where PBC is rare. This is supported by the observation of an increased frequency of urinary tract infections (usually coliform bacteria) in the patients. Nonetheless, no single organism has yet been definitively implicated in the disease.

BIOCHEMICAL LIVER TESTS
In PBC the biochemical tests show a cholestatic pattern of abnormalities, with elevated ALP, GGT and bilirubin but only mildly raised plasma aminotransferases in the earlier stages of the disease. Both the conjugated and unconjugated fractions of bilirubin are elevated. However, a raised ALP in isolation may be the only abnormality in the early stages and cases of asymptomatic PBC have been diagnosed following this finding on routine health screening. The plasma bilirubin concentration is a useful prognostic indicator increasing slowly over the course of the disease and may become very high (> 400 μmol/L) in the later stages. Hypercholesterolaemia is common in PBC, especially early in the course of the disease. Hepatic synthetic function is generally well preserved; the INR is usually normal and, as in cirrhosis of any aetiology, hypoalbuminaemia is seen mainly in patients with long-standing and end-stage disease.

The hypergammaglobulinaemia in PBC is characteristically due to markedly increased plasma IgM concentrations and this is one of the distinguishing features from AIH and PSC. As noted above, patients with PBC have a defect in switching from an IgM to an IgG response following exogenous antigen challenge as well as defective suppression of IgM production. The combination of these two abnormalities (which may be two sides of the same coin) probably accounts for the high IgM concentrations in these patients. Plasma IgA concentrations may be slightly increased but are usually normal, which is a major distinction from alcoholic liver disease (Chapter 5).

AUTOANTIBODIES

ANTIMITOCHONDRIAL ANTIBODIES (AMA)

AMAs represent a broad group of autoantibodies that react with several different antigens in mitochondria. Most sub-specificities of AMA are associated with particular diseases, including some without liver involvement. AMAs are routinely detected by indirect immunofluorescence on unfixed cryostat sections of rat kidney, liver and stomach, giving characteristic staining of mitochondria in the distal renal tubular epithelial cells, in hepatocytes and in gastric parietal cells. At least nine distinct AMAs have been identified, which have been classified as M1 - M9 according to their antigen specificities and disease associations (Figure 6.3). Experienced observers may be able to distinguish between some of the different AMAs according to their immunofluorescent staining patterns but more precise techniques (RIAs, ELISAs, immunoblotting) using the purified target antigens are usually required to discriminate between the various specificities. The M2, M4, M8 and M9 antibodies occur in PBC, but the M2 antibody is the most specific for this disease. M2 reacts with epitopes in the E2 components of the pyruvate dehydrogenase complex (PDC) and other 2-oxo acid dehydrogenases. The antibody is virtually pathognomonic of PBC. It occurs in > 90% of patients with this condition and is usually present at high titres which tend to rise as the disease progresses and persist even after liver transplantation. Also, the majority of apparently healthy individuals who are discovered to have M2 AMA on routine screening are found to have PBC on further investigation. This finding was largely responsible for recognition that PBC has a prolonged asymptomatic phase and that, apparently, some patients may never become symptomatic - indicating that the disease can vary widely in severity. The 2-oxo acid dehydrogenases are located at the bases of the cristae of the inner mitochondrial membranes and why these patients have autoantibodies against such a highly sequestered antigen remains an enigma. However, the E2 epitopes recognised by M2 are highly conserved phylogenetically and can be found in almost all living cells (including yeasts and bacteria), which provides additional support for the impression that an infectious agent may be involved in PBC.

OTHER ANTIBODIES

ANA and/or SMA occur in about 30% of PBC patients at titres >1:40 but pANCA is rare. The SMA react with a variety of cytoskeletal components but, in contrast to AIH, only occasionally with F-actin. The reactivities of ANA in PBC span the whole range of antigen specificities and immunofluorescent staining patterns described earlier. However, three specificities have been recently described that are of particular interest. Two of these relate to ANAs that give the so-called 'nuclear dot' (or speckled) staining pattern on nuclei. Their target antigens have been identified as: i) Sp100, a 53 kDa protein that seems to be partly related to class I HLA molecules, and ii) PML, a nuclear matrix-associated protein with structural features of transcriptional regulatory proteins. The third is an antibody associated with peripheral nuclear staining which reacts with a 210 kDa nuclear pore glycoprotein, Gp210. Detection of these specificities by immunofluorescence can be difficult because staining due to ANAs of other specificities often obscures the specific patterns. Accordingly, demonstration of the specific reactivities usually requires immunoblotting or ELISAs with recombinant proteins or synthetic peptides corresponding to the specific target antigens. Antibodies against these three nuclear antigens occur in 20-30% of PBC patients, including the small proportion who do not have anti-mitochondrial antibodies, and are not found in other liver diseases.

Antimitochondrial antibodies (AMA)	
AMA subtype	**Associated disorders**
M1	Secondary syphilis
M2	Primary biliary cirrhosis
M3	Drug-induced pseudo-lupus syndrome
M4	PBC/AIH 'overlap' cases
M5	Some SLE patients
M6	Some drug-induced hepatitis cases
M7	Various cardiomyopathies
M8	Primary biliary cirrhosis
M9	Primary biliary cirrhosis + some healthy subjects

Figure 6.3   Disease associations of various antimitochondrial autoantibodies (AMA)

HISTOLOGY
Primary biliary cirrhosis is a granulomatous disease in which the classic histological picture is of a well defined granuloma surrounding a damaged bile duct. The

inflammatory infiltrate is comprised predominantly of activated CD4+ and CD8+ lymphocytes - the latter often being seen in contiguity with (and appearing to invade) damaged bile ducts, suggesting that cytotoxic T lymphocytes (CTLs) have a role to play in tissue damage in this condition. Interface hepatitis of varying severity (similar to that seen in AIH) is also often evident, particularly in the earlier stages of the disease.

PRIMARY SCLEROSING CHOLANGITIS

PSC is a disorder that can present at any age and it can be particularly difficult to diagnose in children, who often present with features more suggestive of AIH. Liver histology does not always reveal the characteristic morphological changes of PSC and cholangiography is usually required for a definitive diagnosis. As with PBC, there is uncertainty about whether PSC is truly an autoimmune disease. Hypergammaglobulinaemia and circulating autoantibodies are frequently seen in PSC and the condition is associated with inheritance of the truncated HLA haplo-type B8-DR3. It is also strongly associated with inflammatory bowel disease (IBD). Approximately 70% of patients have IBD, of whom about 85% have ulcerative colitis and 15% have Crohn's disease, although the incidence of PSC in IBD is thought to be less than 5%. Other evidence that provides some support for the concept that it is an autoimmune disease includes the finding that, as in PBC, patients have circulating T lymphocytes that appear to recognise normal biliary tract antigens in vitro. However, in contrast to most autoimmune disorders (including AIH and PBC), there is a male preponderance (M:F ratio > 2:1) in PSC and other data suggest that the disease may be due to chronic bacterial infection of the biliary tract leading to an ascending cholangitis.

BIOCHEMICAL LIVER TESTS
Biochemical abnormalities in PSC usually show a cholestatic pattern, with raised ALP and GGT activities. However, the ALP is usually not elevated to the same extent as in PBC and there have been reports of PSC diagnosed by cholangiog-raphy in patients with normal ALP activities. In the early stages of the disease, bilirubin concentrations are usually normal but these gradually increase (occasion-ally, with striking transient elevations) as the disease progresses. Mild to moderate elevations (less than three times the upper reference limit) of plasma aminotrans-ferase activities are seen in most patients.

The hypergammaglobulinaemia in PSC is due mainly to elevations in plasma IgG concentrations, but it is polyclonal and modest increases in the concentrations of IgM and IgA are also seen. Hepatic synthetic function is usually well preserved until the very late stages following development of cirrhosis but hypoalbu-minaemia may be seen earlier in patients with active IBD. As in other chronic cholestatic liver diseases, concentrations of hepatic and urinary copper and plasma caeruloplasmin are usually increased.

AUTOANTIBODIES

pANCA is the autoantibody most frequently found in the sera of patients with PSC. It occurs at high titres in 65-90% of cases and, in the context of liver disease, was once thought to be a specific marker of this condition. However, the subsequent finding that pANCA occurs with similar frequency in AIH has reduced its diagnostic value in PSC. Between 20% and 30% of PSC patients also have ANA and/or SMA at titres > 1:40 but AMA are almost never observed and, if found, must cast doubt on the diagnosis. Plasma autoantibodies reacting with colonic mucosa are found in up to 65% of PSC patients who have concomitant IBD, compared with about 20% of IBD patients without PSC. However anti-colon antibodies are almost never seen in PSC patients without IBD.

HISTOLOGY

In PSC, the typical morphology is that of a fibrotic lesion, with concentric rings of fibrosis ('onion ring fibrosis') surrounding damaged bile ducts, a mild to moderate inflammatory infiltrate confined to the portal tracts and copper and/or copper-associated protein accumulation in periportal areas. However, as noted above, liver histology may not be diagnostic in the early stages of the disease. Furthermore, as in PBC, portal and periportal lymphoplasmacytic inflammatory activity similar to the interface hepatitis associated with AIH can often be seen at various stages.

OVERLAPPING SYNDROMES

Features of AIH, particularly elevations in plasma IgG, the autoantibodies and HLA markers, and interface hepatitis on liver biopsy, can be seen with variable frequency and/or severity in a wide range of other liver disorders including acute and chronic viral hepatitis (Chapter 3), PBC, PSC, Wilson disease (Chapter 4) and alcoholic liver disease (Chapter 5). This presents problems for diagnosis and, consequently, for clinical management. Corticosteroids are the treatment of choice in AIH and will often reduce parenchymal inflammation in these overlapping conditions, but are usually contraindicated. For example, both PBC and PSC predispose to the development of osteoporosis which can be exacerbated by corticosteroids. Also, steroids enhance viral replication in patients with chronic hepatitis B or C, leading to flares in activity of these diseases when treatment is stopped. On the other hand, interferon (which is currently the most effective treatment for chronic viral hepatitis) can seriously exacerbate underlying autoimmune conditions, particularly AIH and thyroid disease.

The frequency of autoantibodies in chronic hepatitis B and C varies widely in different reports but, overall, significant titres (> 1:40) of ANA and/or SMA occur in 20-40% of cases. Anti-LKM1 is generally very rare in these two conditions but has been reported in up to 6% of patients with chronic hepatitis C in southern Europe. pANCA also seems to be very rare in chronic viral and may be useful for distinguishing between patients with ANA/SMA-positive AIH and those with viral hepatitis who have features of AIH. In this latter group, recent evidence indicates that it is generally safe to use interferon therapy but most authorities agree that careful monitoring of biochemical liver tests, plasma immunoglobulin concentrations and titres of autoantibodies (including thyroid antibodies) is required.

Cholestatic liver disorders with features of AIH have been variously described as: AIH/PBC overlap, AMA-negative PBC, AMA-positive AIH, 'cholestatic AIH' and AIH/PSC overlap. All of these disparate syndromes (if, indeed, they are all distinct) have also been described as 'autoimmune cholangitis' or 'autoimmune cholangiopathy' by different authorities at various times but there is still no universal agreement on the definition of these terms or classification of these conditions. They have three features of AIH in common with each other: elevated plasma IgG (with or without raised IgM), ANA and/or SMA, and histological evidence of interface hepatitis of varying severity (in addition to any biliary changes). They differ with respect to the presence or absence of AMA and whether or not there is also histological evidence of bile duct damage and, if so, whether this is suggestive of either PBC or PSC.

Overlaps with PBC (i.e., AIH/PBC and AMA-negative PBC) are the most common, with up to 30-40% of patients with typical PBC histology having circu-lating ANA and/or SMA and/or some degree of interface hepatitis on liver biopsy. The consensus opinion is that patients with histological evidence of PBC should be included within the spectrum of this disease rather than that of AIH, regardless of whether they have other features suggestive of AIH. Furthermore, recent evidence suggests that the small minority of PBC patients who are AMA seronegative by immunofluorescence have anti-PDC antibodies that react with different epitopes to those of the typical M2 antibodies. Thus it seems likely that few if any PBC patients lack anti-PDC. Similarly, given that AMA (and particularly the M2 subtype) are virtually pathognomonic of PBC, the available evidence suggests that it is likely that most patients with so-called 'AMA-positive AIH' probably have PBC and that failure to find histological changes compatible with PBC is due to early stage of the disease and/or to sampling error on liver biopsy.

'Cholestatic AIH' is a term that is used to describe the 10% or so of AIH patients who present with ALP activities greater than 3x the upper reference interval together with markedly elevated GGT activities without histological evidence of biliary disease. It is possible that some may be occult cases of 'AMA-negative PBC' but this seems unlikely because long-term follow-up of such cases has shown that, in contrast to PBC, they all respond to immunosuppressive therapy with return of the cholestatic indices to normal and no evidence of development of biliary disease.

Overlaps between AIH and PSC are well recognised - particularly in children. In adults, mild to moderate elevations of plasma IgG can be found in about 60%, significant titres of ANA and/or SMA in 20%, HLA B8-DR3 or DR4 in up to 65% and interface hepatitis on liver biopsy in 30-40%. However, only a small minority (about 2%) have combinations of these features with sufficient severity to qualify for a diagnosis of 'definite' AIH. Conversely, there are documented cases (especially in children) of patients presenting with what appears to be AIH but whose disease progresses to clear-cut PSC, sometimes over several years. Due to the rarity of these cases, there is still uncertainty about clinical management. However, many do seem to respond to corticosteroid therapy in terms of resolution of the parenchymal liver damage although the biliary lesions continue to progress.

FURTHER READING

Autoimmune Liver Diseases. Krawitt EL, Wiesner RH, Nishioka M, eds. 2nd ed. Elsevier, Amsterdam; 1998.

Molecular Basis of Autoimmune Hepatitis. McFarlane IG, Williams R, eds. R.G. Landes Co., Austin, Texas; 1996.

Gershwin ME, Mackay IR, eds. Primary biliary cirrhosis. Sem Liv Dis, 1997; **17 (Parts 1 & 2):** 1158.

Lee Y-M, Kaplan MM. Primary sclerosing cholangitis. New Engl J Med, 1995; **332:** 924-33.

Chapter 7

Hepatic malignancies

INTRODUCTION

As with all tumours, those affecting the liver can be classified as benign or malig-nant, the latter being further sub-classified as primary or secondary. Primary hepatic tumours may arise from any of the cell types in the liver: hepatocellular carcinoma (HCC) from the hepatocytes, cholangiocarcinoma from the cells of the bile ducts, and hepatic sarcoma from the endothelial cells. The liver is the commonest site for metastatic deposits from primary tumours arising elsewhere in the body. In the Western world, primary liver cancer is relatively rare and patients with secondary hepatic malignancy outnumber those with primary tumours by about 50:1. In parts of sub-Saharan Africa and in the Middle and Far East, however, primary HCC is much more common. The wide geographical variation in the incidence of HCC is probably related to differences in the prevalence of hepatitis B and C carriage between countries, for this, together with chronic liver disease (particularly cirrhosis), is the main aetiological factor in the development of HCC. Hepatocellular carcinoma is a highly malignant tumour and patients seldom survive more than one year from the onset of symptoms.

Apart from the fact that the likelihood of significant hepatic malignancy is low if the plasma activities of the liver enzymes (AST, ALT, ALP, GGT) and the bilirubin concentration are within their reference ranges, the standard liver biochemistry tests are of little value in the diagnosis of liver tumours as the abnormalities observed are non-specific. In a patient in whom hepatic malignancy is suspected, imaging techniques such as ultrasound, hepatic angiography or CT scanning are usually used to identify the presence and location of a lesion, whilst histological examination of biopsy specimens is required to confirm the diagnosis. A simple serological test which allows confident diagnosis and accurate monitoring of therapy is a long-sought goal of the oncologist and the knowledge that some tumours synthesise and secrete substances that have some degree of specificity towards particular tumours has led to the investigation of many potential substances as tumour markers.

The ideal tumour marker would be one that is :

- easily and reliably detected in plasma,
- specific to a certain histological type of tumour,
- sufficiently sensitive to detect all cases of that tumour,

- detectable at an early stage of tumour development when treatment may be effective,
- has a plasma concentration proportional to the viable cell mass of the tumour, in order to permit the accurate monitoring of therapy.

To date, no such perfect test has been devised for any tumour, but in primary liver tumours α-fetoprotein (AFP) for HCC and CA 19-9 for cholangiocarcinoma and other biliary tract malignancies are of some value. Tumour markers are of little value in the diagnosis of secondary hepatic malignancy.

α-FETOPROTEIN

AFP is by far the most important serological tumour marker in hepatology. It is a glycopeptide with a molecular weight of about 72 kDa and is composed of 590 amino acids with a complex arrangement of carbohydrate side chains. Several isoforms exist, differing with respect to their carbohydrate moieties, which may prove to be useful diagnostically. AFP was first detected in 1963 in mice with chemically induced liver tumours and in a patient with HCC the following year. It was defined as an oncofetal protein but its specific function is not known. AFP shares many characteristics with albumin having an overall sequence homology of about 40% and it may be its embryonic analogue.

In the fetus, AFP is normally synthesised in large amounts only by the yolk sac, liver and gut. By the third month of gestation, fetal plasma concentrations of AFP rise to 2000-3000 µg/L and thereafter fall progressively as albumin synthesis proceeds and the volume of distribution increases. In the mother, plasma AFP concentrations rise from about 30 µg/L at 16 weeks gestation to about 500 µg/L at term. Plasma AFP concentrations at birth span a wide range but fall progressively to about 30 µg/L at one month and reach the normal adult range of 0-10 µg/L by about one year of life (Figure 7.1). In HCC, AFP appears to be produced solely by the malignant cells as there is no evidence of reactive synthesis by surrounding normal hepatocytes. Plasma concentrations of AFP in HCC may reach 1 g/L and as the actual value is of prognostic significance it is important that samples be appropriately diluted to determine the precise concentration. It is equally important with immunometric assays for AFP that the concentration at which the 'hook-effect' becomes significant is known.

DIAGNOSIS OF HCC IN THE SYMPTOMATIC PATIENT

Plasma AFP concentrations are elevated in about 80% of patients with symptomatic HCC overall, but are only occasionally increased in patients with metastatic liver disease and are almost always normal in other types of primary liver tumours. However, this frequency falls to about 50% in patients with HCC who do not have cirrhosis. Repeated AFP measurement in patients with a normal AFP but definite HCC is of no value, because if a particular tumour does not secrete AFP at presentation it will not do so during the subsequent course of the disease, i.e., AFP-negative tumours do not become AFP-positive tumours and vice versa.

Plasma AFP from birth to adulthood		
Age	**Number**	**Mean ± S.D. (µg/L)**
Premature	11	134,700 ± 41,500
Newborn	55	48,400 ± 34,700
Newborn - 2 weeks	16	33,100 ± 32,500
2 weeks - 1 month	43	9,450 ± 12,600
1 m	12	2,650 ± 3,080
2 m	40	323 ± 278
3 m	5	88 ± 87
4 m	31	74 ± 56
5 m	6	46 ± 19
6 m	9	12.5 ± 9.8
> 6 m	8	8.5 ± 5.5

Figure 7.1 Upper reference limits for serum AFP from birth to adulthood

Patients with uncomplicated cirrhosis may occasionally have plasma AFP concentrations up to 100 µg/L without any evidence of HCC and patients with untreated chronic hepatitis (with or without cirrhosis) can also, occasionally, have concentrations as high as 500 µg/L. This presents a real diagnostic problem as the development of HCC is a definite possibility in a cirrhotic patient with clinical deterioration (e.g., accumulation of ascites). A plasma AFP concentration greater than 500 µg/L is virtually diagnostic of HCC but lower values are harder to interpret, although a rising AFP on serial measurement should produce a high index of suspicion of malignancy. Similarly, in a patient without cirrhosis in whom the differential diagnosis includes primary or secondary liver tumours, a plasma AFP concentration of more than 500 µg/L effectively confirms HCC but as 50% of such patients have a normal AFP, a negative result is of little value.

Other conditions in which elevated plasma concentrations of AFP are found include acute hepatic failure, in which the AFP is often raised (occasionally as high as 1000 µg/L). Minor elevations of AFP are also often seen in the later stages of uncomplicated acute viral hepatitis but concentrations rarely exceed 100 µg/L. Neither of these conditions should cause any diagnostic confusion, for HCC does not usually enter the differential diagnosis of patients presenting with acute hepatitic illnesses. It should be noted that other primary tumours may secrete AFP, including germ cell tumours and tumours of the pancreas, stomach and gall bladder regardless of whether they have metastasised to the liver.

SCREENING FOR HCC IN THE ASYMPTOMATIC PATIENT
Despite the specificity of a markedly elevated plasma AFP concentration for HCC, it is not worthwhile (on clinical or economical grounds) to screen large populations of patients who are at low risk of developing this tumour. It may, however, be more fruitful to screen high risk groups (such as hepatitis B and C carriers or patients with cirrhosis) in whom the HCC detection rate could be as high as 5 per 1000 patients tested.

As noted above, the finding of an AFP concentration of greater than 500 µg/L in a cirrhotic patient is virtually diagnostic of HCC whereas a value between 50 and 500 µg/L warrants more detailed investigation, both by repeating the test to detect a rising level and by imaging techniques. There is no doubt that, if patients with cirrhosis are regularly screened at intervals of 3 to 6 months, a diagnosis of HCC can be established months or years before clinical symptoms develop. Given the poor prognosis in HCC, whether or not this is of advantage to the patient is another matter. There is, however, some evidence that there is a lower recurrence rate for HCC following liver transplantation in patients in whom the diagnosis is established before clinical symptoms develop. In high-incidence areas, particularly China, other parts of the Far East and in Alaska, mass screening programmes combining plasma AFP and ultrasound have been instituted and have led to the early detection of tumours. It appears that in these areas tumours may develop when cirrhosis is at a less advanced stage and there is a greater chance that they can be successfully resected. The AFP concentrations found in patients with these smaller, presymptomatic tumours are generally lower than in symptomatic patients.

ROLE OF AFP MEASUREMENTS IN THE MANAGEMENT OF HCC

Serial AFP measurements can be valuable for monitoring the response to treatment (chemotherapy, resection, arterial embolization or transplantation) in patients with AFP-positive HCC. Although the intra-individual variation in plasma AFP concentrations for a given tumour cell mass is wide, for a given patient the concentration usually varies in proportion to tumour mass and will increase exponentially (with a doubling time of approximately 40 days) in the absence of treatment. With surgical removal of the tumour, plasma AFP concentrations fall to within the reference range with a half-life of about four days. This should not, however, be taken to indicate that all of the tumour has been removed as it seems that there is a minimum threshold mass of tumour that is required to produce sufficient AFP to exceed the upper reference limit in plasma. In this situation, the plasma AFP concentrations should be monitored monthly for several months as rising concentrations would indicate tumour regrowth. (Figure 7.2)

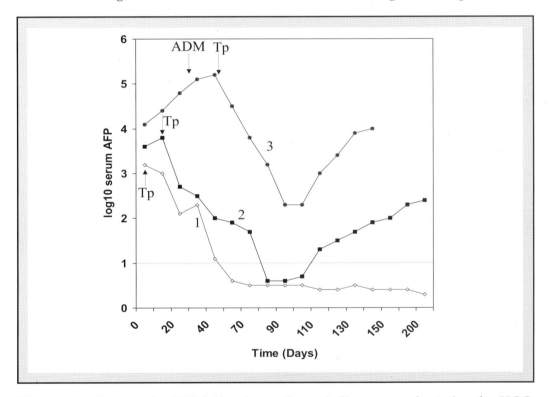

Figure 7.2 Changes in AFP following orthotopic liver transplantation for HCC. There was no macroscopic evidence of tumour after operation in any patient. Patient 1 remains well 10 years after transplantation. Patient 2 showed subsequent recurrence despite having achieved normal AFP concentrations. patient 3 did not achieve normal AFP concentrations at any time suggesting residual tumour

The fall in plasma AFP concentrations following effective chemotherapy can be exploited to optimise therapy. A decrease in plasma AFP over the initial 1–2 months of treatment indicates the drug is effective (Figure 7.3), whereas a continued rise in plasma AFP indicates that the tumour is persistent and another drug or course of therapy substituted. This approach avoids prolonged chemotherapy without benefit, thereby reducing toxicity.

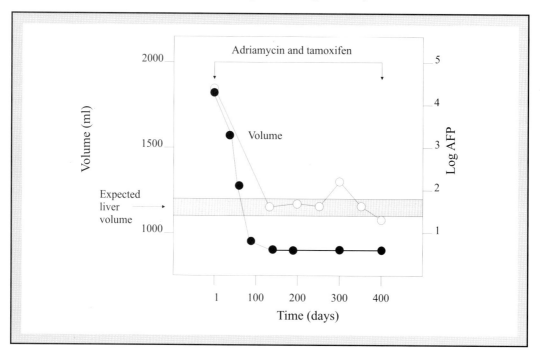

Figure 7.3 Changes in AFP following cytotoxic chemotherapy. This patient underwent complete clinical remission. Plasma AFP fell in parallel with the decreasing liver volume as measured by ultrasound examination

It should be noted that, while there is no direct relationship between plasma AFP (either its presence or absence or absolute concentration) and prognosis, patients with normal or only slowly rising plasma AFP concentrations tend to survive longer. Patients with relentlessly increasing plasma AFP despite chemotherapy have a poor prognosis.

AFP IN PAEDIATRIC LIVER DISEASE
Grossly elevated plasma AFP concentrations are seen in virtually all children with hepatoblastoma and in about 75% with HCC. However, neonatal hepatitis of any cause is also associated with abnormal plasma AFP concentrations and this makes interpretation difficult in the first year of life. Other childhood disorders in which

high plasma AFP concentrations may be found include tyrosinaemia and the ataxia telangiectasia syndrome

AFP MICROHETEROGENEITY

The range of plasma AFP concentrations between 10 and 500 µg/L constitutes a grey area for interpretation as the specificity for HCC is poor. Apart from the use of serial testing, interest has focused on observations that some tumours may produce AFP with a different carbohydrate side chain composition to that normally seen. Initial work utilised differences in the binding of plasma AFP from patients with HCC to concanavalin A and lentil lectins compared with that of AFP from patients with cirrhosis but no tumour. Subsequently isoelectric focusing has demonstrated that differences in the isoform composition can occur before the total concentration reaches a diagnostically useful level (Figure 7.4). Two isoforms (AFP III and IV), with isoelectric points more alkaline than the dominant form, are strongly associated with HCC. These isoforms are present in approximately 80% of patients with HCC but less than 15% of patients with non-malignant liver disease. In some patients the isoforms have been detected many months prior to elevations of total AFP and before the tumour can be detected by ultrasound.

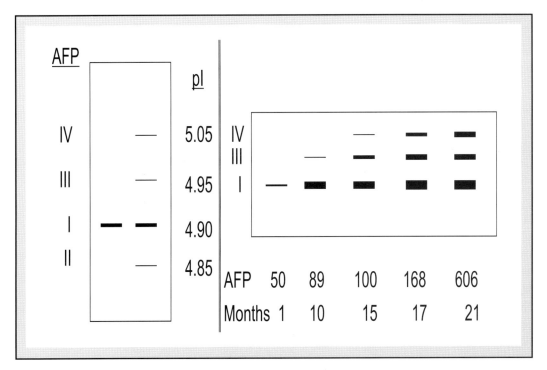

Figure 7.4 Microheterogeneity of AFP in HCC. The isoforms III and IV are present prior to recurrence of tumour in this patient at 21 months following initial surgery

OTHER PLASMA MARKERS OF HEPATOCELLULAR CARCINOMA

Many plasma components have been investigated as potential tumour markers for HCC including a variant of GGT, des-gamma-carboxy prothrombin, alkaline phosphatase isoenzymes and the vitamin B12 binding proteins. However, only the latter two have found their way into routine use.

ALKALINE PHOSPHATASE

A variant isoenzyme of alkaline phosphatase has been observed in up to 30% of cases of HCC. It appears to be equivalent to the fetal intestinal isoenzyme and is sometimes called the Kasahara isoenzyme. It is not known why some hepatoma cells re-express a foetal isoenzyme but its presence in plasma is highly specific for HCC although sensitivity is low with only 5-30% of tumours producing it. The isoenzyme can be detected by the routine gel electrophoresis method used for alkaline phosphatase isoenzymes where it runs as a fast moving band ahead of the main liver band. This isoenzyme is distinct from the placental isoenzyme which is detectable in the sera of up to 10% of patients with various non-hepatic primary tumours.

VITAMIN B12 BINDING PROTEINS

Vitamin B12 (cobalamin) is transported in the circulation by the binding proteins known as transcobalamins. Abnormalities of cobalamin metabolism have been reported in HCC patients, with the plasma concentrations of transcobalamins I and III (two proteins differing only in their sialic acid composition) being markedly higher compared with patients with non-malignant liver disease. Particularly high concentrations of the transcobalamins are seen in the rare histological variant of HCC, fibrolamellar carcinoma, and can be used to monitor treatment in these cases.

TUMOUR MARKERS IN BILIARY TRACT MALIGNANCIES

Cholangiocarcinoma was originally described in association with ulcerative colitis but it is now generally believed that these patients had concomitant primary sclerosing cholangitis (PSC). PSC is a progressive condition with over half the symptomatic patients eventually progressing to severe hepatic failure. At present, liver transplantation is the only effective treatment but this is complicated by the high incidence (up to 40%) of cholangiocarcinoma in PSC patients which often recurs post-transplant. Regular monitoring of PSC patients is therefore required to optimise the timing of liver transplantation. Ultrasonography, CT scanning and endoscopic retrograde cholangiopancreatography (ERCP) have relatively low sensitivity for the detection of cholangiocarcinoma and are expensive for repetitive testing. A combination of the serological tumour markers CEA and CA19-9 has been found to be of value in identifying cholangiocarcinoma in PSC patients.

CA19-9 is the antigen target of a monoclonal antibody 116NS19-9 obtained from mice infected with the human colonic carcinoma cell line SW1116. It is a sialylated Lewis A blood group antigen: sialosyl-fucosyl-lactotetraose. CA19-9 is expressed on the cell surfaces of the biliary and pancreatic duct cells and in some cells in the colon. CA19-9 is now the tumour marker of choice in pancreatic cancer, but grossly elevated plasma CA19-9 concentrations have been observed in biliary tract obstruction either from gall stones or from primary biliary cancer. CA19-9 has been shown to increase in plasma in PSC in proportion to disease activity and can be useful in monitoring patients with a view to undertaking liver transplantation prior to the onset of acute hepatic failure. If cholangiocarcinoma is present, plasma CA19-9 rises sharply and very high concentrations (>10,000 kU/L) can be seen. CEA, on the other hand remains normal in PSC but is often, though not invariably, raised when cholangiocarcinoma is present. A combined index of the two markers (CA19-9 + (CEA x 40)) has been derived which can give an accuracy of up to 85% for the diagnosis of cholangiocarcinoma in PSC (Figure 7.5). It must, however, be noted that individuals whose blood group is Lewis a-b- will not express CA19-9; plasma concentrations will always be below the detection limit of the assay. Additionally, cholestasis can itself cause an increase in plasma CA19-9, limiting the usefulness of the marker in diagnosis.

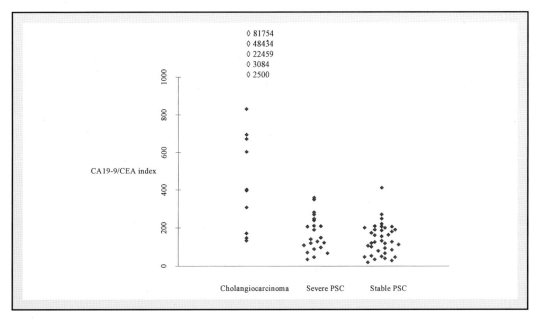

Figure 7.5 Plasma CEA/CA19-9 index in patients with active and stable PSC and in patients with cholangiocarcinoma

TUMOUR MARKERS IN SECONDARY LIVER CANCER

Tumour markers are of far less importance in the diagnosis and management of the more common liver tumours that originate from primary tumours elsewhere. With the notable exception of markers related to carcinoid tumours, CEA is the only plasma marker that is of proven value in secondary liver cancer.

CARCINOEMBRYONIC ANTIGEN

CEA is a glycoprotein with a molecular weight of 200 kDa which is produced in small amounts by the normal gut but in much greater quantities by some colorectal carcinomas. There is considerable variation in the amount of CEA synthesised by cancer cells and the plasma concentrations also depend on the vascularity of the particular tumour. CEA is cleared by the liver and mild elevations in the plasma concentrations can be seen in some benign liver diseases. CEA is not of value as a diagnostic test for colonic carcinoma but has a role in the detection of hepatic metastases in patients who have undergone attempted curative resection of primary tumours. Rapidly rising concentrations, exceeding 40 µg/L within six months of the first positive value, are strongly suggestive of hepatic metastases. Such changes often predate clinical symptoms by up to six months (Figure 7.6) and presumably reflect both the ease of secretion of CEA from the liver into the circulation and possibly diminished clearance as a consequence of hepatocellular damage from the metastases. Plasma CEA is of less value in detecting local recurrence of tumour but a fall in plasma concentration following intra-arterial chemotherapy predicts subsequent clinical response.

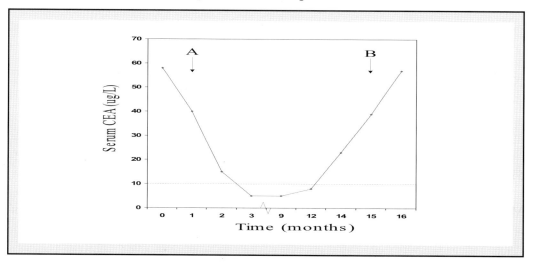

Figure 7.6 Serial CEA measurements following resection of a colonic carcinoma. There was no evidence of hepatic deposits at the time of the initial resection (A), but hepatic tumour could be detected on CT scanning at time B, four months after the CEA concentration began to rise

CARCINOID TUMOURS AND THE CARCINOID SYNDROME

Carcinoid tumours are derived from enterochromaffin cells, which are widely distributed throughout the body. Tumours that originate in the small bowel often produce large quantities of vasoactive peptides, particularly serotonin which is inactivated by the liver. If hepatic metastases develop, serotonin is released into the systemic circulation and causes episodic flushing and diarrhoea - the carcinoid syndrome. Serotonin is produced from tryptophan and is metabolised to 5-hydroxyindoleacetic acid (5-HIAA) which is excreted in the urine. (Figure 7.7)

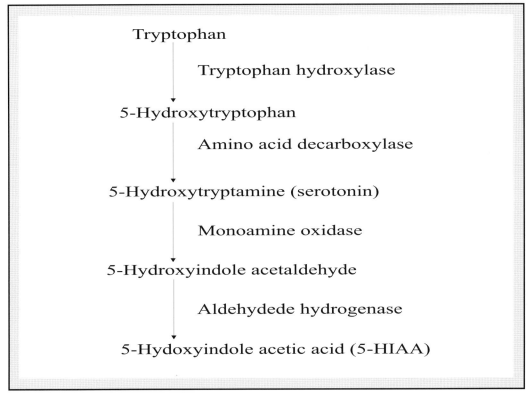

Figure 7.7 Pathway of serotonin metabolism

Measurement of the urinary excretion of 5-HIAA is valuable in the diagnosis of carcinoid tumours and in monitoring therapy. Normally less than 40 µmol of 5-HIAA is excreted in urine per 24h and excretion > 120 µmol/24h is virtually diagnostic of carcinoid. False negative results occur with foregut tumours, which often lack the enzyme amino acid decarboxylase and consequently secrete 5-hydroxytryptophan rather than serotonin. In anuric patients, plasma serotonin measurements can replace urine 5-HIAA. False positive results can be obtained in patients consuming foods rich in serotonin e.g., bananas, pineapples, walnuts and avocados. Mildly elevated 5-HIAA excretion occurs in some patients with coeliac disease due to overproduction of serotonin in the cells of the small intestine. The urinary excretion of 5-HIAA varies proportionately with tumour mass and can be a useful method of monitoring therapy, which is usually occlusion of the hepatic artery by either embolization or ligation (Figure 7.8).

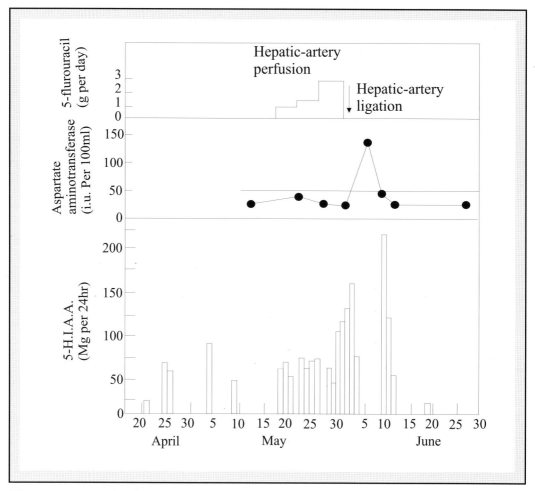

Figure 7.8 Monitoring response of a carcinoid tumour to treatment using serial measurements of urinary 5-HIAA excretion. There was no response to hepatic artery perfusion of the cytotoxic drug 5-fluorouracil, but hepatic artery ligation led to a fall in 5-HIAA to undetectable concentrations. Note the transient rise in AST reflecting tumour necrosis. The patient was symptom free after surgery.

FURTHER READING

Beastall GH, Cook B, Rustin GJS. A review of the role of the established tumour markers. Ann Clin Biochem 1991; **28:** 5-18.

Burditt LJ, Johnson M, Johnson PJ, Williams R. Detection of hepatocellular carcinoma-specific alpha-fetoprotein by isoelectric focusing. Cancer 1994; **74:** 25-9.

Deacon A. The measurement of 5-hydroxy-indoleacetic acid in urine . Ann Clin Biochem 1994; **31:** 215-32.

Fremont S, Champigneulle B, Gerard P, Felden F, Lambert D, Gueant JL, et al. Blood transcobalamin levels in malignant hepatoma. Tumour Biol 1991; **12:** 353-9.

Maestranzi S, Przemioslo R, Mitchell HC, Sherwood R. The effect of benign and malignant liver disease on the tumour markers CA 19-9 and CEA. Ann Clin Biochem. 1998; **35:** 99-103.

Ramage JK, Donaghy A, Farrant JM, Iorns R, Williams R. Serum tumour markers for the diagnosis of cholangiocarcinoma in primary sclerosing cholangitis. Gastroenterology 1995; **108:** 865-9.

Sawahu N, Hattori N. Serological markers in hepatocellular carcinoma. In: Neoplasms of the Liver (Okuda K and Ishak KG, Eds) pp227-37 Tokyo: Springer-Verlag, 1987.

Chapter 8

Pregnancy and Liver Disease

INTRODUCTION

Liver disease in pregnancy is rare, but when it does occur it can be severe with significant risk to both mother and foetus. Improvements in the treatment of liver disease have resulted in women with liver disease, who would previously have been unable to conceive, becoming pregnant and the impact of the pregnancy on their liver disease may present problems in their management. Pre-existing liver disease, often previously undiagnosed, may be exacerbated by pregnancy, particularly primary biliary cirrhosis and also the Dubin-Johnson syndrome which may present with jaundice in the second or third trimester. There are also some liver diseases and other conditions in which hepatic function is altered which are unique to pregnancy. The presenting features, prevalence and the impact of these diseases on the outcome of pregnancy are shown in Figure 8.1.

The normal physiological changes in pregnancy can cause alterations in many of the standard biochemical and haematological indices as well as physical signs which can mimic those seen in liver disease. Plasma albumin concentrations fall due to an increase in plasma volume and can be below the lower limit of the reference range by the third trimester. Similarly, plasma alkaline phosphatase activities rise 2 - 4 fold over the course of pregnancy due to the contribution from the placental isoenzyme leaking into the circulation. In the absence of iron deficiency red cell mass increases by 10-20% during pregnancy, but the increase in plasma volume outweighs this and haemoglobin concentration, haematocrit and red cell count fall to near or below the lower limit of their reference intervals by the third trimester. Changes in the coagulation systems during pregnancy include a reduction in the platelet count and increases in the concentrations of the majority of the clotting factors. Fibrinolytic activity is increased during pregnancy and increased fibrin degradation products occur indicating fibrin formation. Telangiectasia and palmar erythema can be seen in a significant proportion of pregnant women. All of the above changes rapidly return to normal following delivery. Normal pregnancy has only a minimal effect on the plasma activities of the liver enzymes AST, ALT and GGT. Any increase in these enzymes must, therefore, be considered to indicate hepatic pathology. If the effect of pre-existing haemolytic disease such as sickle cell anaemia is excluded, plasma bilirubin concentration also remains within normal limits during pregnancy and can be useful in identifying significant liver disease.

Unlike those diseases such as viral hepatitis, which may occur in both non-pregnant women and pregnant women at any stage of pregnancy, conditions affecting the liver that are specific to pregnancy occur at characteristic times. Hyperemesis gravidum usually occurs in the first trimester whilst intrahepatic cholestasis of pregnancy, acute fatty liver of pregnancy and the related group of conditions, pre-eclampsia, eclampsia and the HELLP syndrome (haemolysis, elevated liver enzymes and low platelet count) all occur later. For convenience, conditions affecting the liver that are specific to pregnancy can be divided into those that are predominantly cholestatic and those in which there is hepatocellular damage. The presenting symptoms and the alterations to the standard biochemical liver tests will usually separate the disease into one of these categories.

Liver disease in pregnancy			
Disease	**Symptoms**	**Trimester**	**Effects on outcome**
Hyperemesis gravidum	Nausea, vomiting	1	Low birth weight if maternal weight loss
Intrahepatic cholestasis of pregnancy	Pruritis	2 or 3	Stillbirth, premature birth
Acute fatty liver of pregnancy	Upper abdominal pain, nausea and vomiting, encephalopathy in late stages	3	Maternal and foetal mortality (10-15%)
Pre-eclampsia/ eclampsia	Hypertension, oedema, proteinuria, headaches, visual disturbances	2 or 3	Increased maternal mortality (1%)
HELLP syndrome	Upper abdominal pain, nausea and vomiting	3	Increased maternal (2%) and foetal (35%) mortality

Figure 8.1 Conditions affecting the liver that are specific to pregnancy

CHOLESTATIC DISEASES IN PREGNANCY

The presenting features of cholestatic liver disease in pregnancy are pruritis (itching) and mild jaundice; abdominal pain is rare. The non-pregnancy specific liver diseases included in the differential diagnosis include primary biliary cirrhosis, drug-induced cholestasis and Dubin-Johnson syndrome. The two conditions unique to pregnancy which cause cholestasis are hyperemesis gravidum (first trimester) and intrahepatic cholestasis of pregnancy (second and third trimesters). Biliary tract disease, caused by gallstones, may occur at any time but is accompanied by pain in the right upper quadrant and fever.

HYPEREMESIS GRAVIDUM

Hyperemesis gravidum generally occurs in the first trimester of pregnancy, but can be seen as late as 20 weeks. It is characterised by nausea and vomiting which can lead acutely to dehydration and chronically to a sub-optimal nutritional status. Jaundice is mild with plasma bilirubin concentration seldom exceeding 75 µmol/L, the increase being in both the conjugated and unconjugated fractions. The mechanism of hyperbilirubinaemia is unclear but may be related to impaired excretion of bilirubin. The aminotransferases are elevated up to 200 IU/L and 2-4 fold elevations in alkaline phosphatase and GGT occur indicating cholestasis. Histologically the liver may show mild fatty change but is otherwise normal. Although the underlying cause of the condition is unknown, the abnormalities in the liver are probably related to malnutrition as if a normal nutrient intake can be restored, the abnormal laboratory test results rapidly return to normal. Hyperemesis gravidum does not usually have major adverse effects on the outcome of the pregnancy, although in severe cases the baby's birth weight may be lower than is usual in milder cases or unaffected pregnancies.

INTRAHEPATIC CHOLESTASIS OF PREGNANCY

This condition was initially described as a syndrome occurring in pregnant Swedish women, but can occur in other populations. Pruritis may be severe and jaundice develops in most cases 1–4 weeks after the onset of itching. Onset is typically in the third trimester but in a small proportion of cases (< 25%) it may be earlier. Symptoms persist until delivery and resolve rapidly thereafter. Features of biliary obstruction are present including bilirubin in the urine and pale stools. Plasma bilirubin concentrations are elevated (up to 100 µmol/L), alkaline phosphatase may be increased up to 4-10 times the reference interval with the hepatic isoenzyme predominating, but aminotransferases activities are variable from normal to values similar to those occurring in viral hepatitis. The rise in the plasma aminotransferases can, however, be transient. The plasma total bile acid concentration is markedly elevated (10-100-fold) and this may occasionally be the only abnormality, so that assay of bile acids can sometimes aid in confirming the diagnosis. Liver histology is unhelpful, as the changes are identical to those in cholestasis from several other causes.

Diagnosis of intrahepatic cholestasis of pregnancy is important, as the condition is associated with an increased risk of premature delivery and stillbirth (up to 3% in some studies). Treatment with cholestyramine may provide some relief from the symptoms and early delivery should be considered. The pathogenesis of the condition is unknown but evidence is mounting for a genetic basis. The prevalence is higher in some populations (Sweden, Chile) and the recurrence rate in subsequent pregnancies can be as high as 70%.

OTHER CAUSES OF CHOLESTASIS DURING PREGNANCY

Pregnant women, particularly those who have previously taken oral contraceptives, have an increased risk of developing gallstones. In many cases, these may not be clinically apparent and there is evidence that they may spontaneously disappear during the first year after delivery. One other condition worthy of note is thrombosis of the hepatic venous (outflow) system, known as the Budd-Chiari syndrome, which has an increased incidence in pregnancy. This usually manifests itself during the immediate post-partum period and is throught to be related to a hypercoagulable state due to lower antithrombin III concentrations at the time of delivery. The foetus is unaffected but maternal mortality due to liver failure is high.

HEPATOCELLULAR LIVER DISEASE IN PREGNANCY

An acute 'hepatic' presentation in the first trimester of pregnancy is more likely to be due to viral infection which must also be considered as part of the differential diagnosis in the later stages of pregnancy. Viral hepatitis has a similar incidence in pregnancy to that in the non-pregnant population and the clinical squelae are also similar, with the exception of hepatitis E. The mortality rate from hepatitis E infection in pregnancy approaches 20% in some regions (e.g., India, Africa and the Middle East). The pregnancy specific liver diseases in this category are acute fatty liver of pregnancy and the group of conditions associated with hypertension, namely pre-eclampsia, eclampsia and the HELLP syndrome. All of these conditions occur in the second and third trimester of pregnancy.

ACUTE FATTY LIVER OF PREGNANCY. (AFLP)

AFLP was first described in 1940 as 'obstetric acute yellow atrophy'. It is characterised histologically by hepatocellular swelling and microvesicular fat infiltration, primarily in the pericentral zone. AFLP is rare before 28 weeks with symptoms typically developing between 33 and 37 weeks gestation. Initial clinical findings are non-specific with nausea and vomiting, upper abdominal pain and a viral-like illness. Jaundice then follows with rapid progression, in untreated cases, to fulminant hepatic failure. The foetal and maternal mortality rate has been reduced substantially in recent years, but is still around 10-20%. As the condition usually resolves after delivery, rapid termination of the pregnancy is often advised. In some cases liver function does not improve post-partum and liver transplantation may become necessary.

Hyperbilirubinaemia is invariable and usually severe with a rise primarily in conjugated bilirubin. Plasma alkaline phosphatase and the aminotransferases are elevated, markedly so in a proportion of cases. Hypoglycaemia is often present. There is evidence of disseminated intravascular coagulopathy in up to 50% of cases. Hyperuricaemia may also be present and a number of patients have been reported to have hypertension, leading to speculation that AFLP may be linked to pre-eclampsia. However, half of the patients with AFLP never have hypertension and most cases of pre-eclampsia that progress, do so to eclampsia or the HELLP syndrome rather than to AFLP. Recently, several cases of AFLP have been reported in which the foetus has been affected by a fatty acid oxidation defect and it has been suggested that this may be a causal factor in the development of AFLP in the mother. Although initially considered to be a rare condition, AFLP is now thought to have an incidence of 1 in 13,000 pregnancies, a figure similar to that for the combined fatty acid oxidation defects.

PRE-ECLAMPSIA, ECLAMPSIA AND THE HELLP SYNDROME

Pre-eclampsia is characterised by the development of hypertension, proteinuria and oedema late in the second or in the third trimester. The American College of Obstetricians and Gynaecologists has defined pregnancy-induced hypertension as an increase of 30 mmHg (systolic) or 15 mmHg (diastolic) above the equivalent value in the first trimester or a blood pressure above 140/90 at any time. Pre-eclampsia may present with visual disturbances or headaches or be detected by proteinuria or hyperuricaemia. It complicates approximately 5% of pregnancies, occuring more frequently in women with pre-existing hypertension, in first pregnancies and with twin/triplet pregnancies. The nearer to term the onset of pre-eclampsia, the better the outcome is for both mother and foetus. Maternal mortality has now been reduced to less than 1% at most centres with death usually due to central nervous system or hepatic complications. Eclampsia is the more severe stage of pre-eclampsia with blood pressures greater than 160/90, gross proteinuria (> 5 g/24h), seizures and coma. The HELLP syndrome is a further complication of severe pre-eclampsia/eclampsia.

The diagnosis of pre-eclampsia is based on the findings of hypertension and proteinuria, with or without oedema; other laboratory tests are often normal at this stage. The plasma aminotransferases and uric acid rise in proportion to disease severity reflecting the degree of hepatocellular damage that is occurring. In women with severe pre-eclampsia it is estimated that 5-10% may develop the HELLP syndrome acutely, with abdominal pain, nausea and vomiting and prolonged bleeding being the most common symptoms. In the HELLP syndrome there is evidence of a disseminated intravascular coagulopathy. The platelet count is usually < 100 x 10^9/L, plasma concentrations of fibrinogen and antithrombin III are reduced with increased levels of fibrin degradation products and a prolonged INR. Plasma liver enzyme activities are invariably raised but are seldom more than 1000 IU/L. Hyperbilirubinaemia is usually moderate and predominantly involves the unconjugated fraction, reflecting intravascular haemolysis which results in anaemia as the disease progresses. Apart from the haemolysis and low platelet count there are other features which distinguish the HELLP syndrome from AFLP: in AFLP the liver is often small, there is an elevated white cell count (> 15 x 10^9/L) and, hyperammonaemia occurs together with hepatic encephalopathy. None of these features are present in the HELLP syndrome.

The mortality rate for women with HELLP is approximately 2-3%. Complications include placental abruption, renal failure and pulmonary oedema associated with congestive cardiac failure. The perinatal mortality can be up to 35%. Delivery is the only effective treatment. Infants are, therefore, at risk of the complications of prematurity and additionally can develop thrombocytopaenia. In up to one quarter of patients, the condition may occur in subsequent pregnancies.

The pathogenesis of pre-eclampsia is unclear but the underlying hypertension is presumably a consequence of inappropriate vasoconstriction. Various hypotheses have been put forward to account for this phenomenon. In particular, a role for prostaglandins has been suggested. Thromboxane A2, produced primarily by platelets, is a potent vasoconstrictor the action of which may be balanced by the vasodilatory effects of prostacyclin. It has been proposed that endothelial cell damage leads to reduced prostacyclin production, as the vascular endothelium is the primary site of this process. This leads to an imbalance in the thromboxane A2:prostacyclin ratio, promoting vasoconstriction and consequent hypertension. Aspirin taken prophylactically in the third trimester of pregnancy by women at high risk of pre-eclampsia appears to lower the incidence of the condition, a finding which would support the involvement of prostaglandins: aspirin inhibits thromboxane production but has minimal effects on prostacyclin metabolism. The observation that plasma fibronectin concentrations are higher in women who subsequently developed pre-eclampsia compared with normal values in pregnancy lends further support to the suggestion that endothelial damage is important in the pathogenesis of pre-eclampsia. An alternative hypothesis is the involvement of immunological mechanisms. This possibility is indirectly supported by the observation of a higher incidence of pre-eclampsia in primigravidae and following paternal change. No firm evidence of immunological abnormalities has, however, yet been found to support this theory.

PREGNANCY AND PRE-EXISTING LIVER DISEASE

Women with advanced liver disease are often amenorrheic and do not ovulate, and therefore seldom become pregnant. The amenorrhea is thought to be due to hypothalamic-pituitary dysfunction and is not directly related to the severity of the liver disease. Nonetheless, pregnancies do occur, and the frequency is increasing with improvements in clinical management of patients with liver disease. Pregnancy can be sustained without worsening of hepatic function and foetal abnormalities are rare, but there is a slightly increased incidence of miscarriages and premature deliveries. In any patient with liver disease, however, careful monitoring during pregnancy is required.

Pregnancy should be avoided in patients with cirrhosis complicated by portal hypertension and gastric or oesophageal varices. Because of the increase in intra-abdominal pressure in the mother as the foetus develops, there is a great risk in such cases of exacerbation of the portal hypertension and variceal rupture.

In younger female recipients of liver transplants, the normal menstrual pattern returns quickly after operation and there are now many reports of successful pregnancies in such women. Ideally pregnancy should be deferred for at least one year following liver transplantation. Women with autoimmune hepatitis similarly find that they begin to ovulate again when their disease enters remission and, indeed, often become pregnant without being aware of the return of their fertility. In most such cases, pregnancy is normal but about 25% experience relapses of their disease during pregnancy or shortly after delivery.

FURTHER READING

Barron W. The syndrome of pre-eclampsia. Gastroenterol Clin North Am 1992; **21:** 851-72.

Barton JR, Sibai BM. Care of the pregnancy complicated by HELLP syndrome. Gastroenterol Clin North Am 1992; **21:** 937-50.

Freund G, Arvan DA. Clinical biochemistry of pre-eclampsia and related liver diseases in pregnancy: a review. Clin Chim Acta 1990; **191:** 123-52.

Friedman SA. Pre-eclampsia: A review of the role of prostaglandins. Obstet Gynaecol 1988; **71:** 122-37.

Knox TA, Olans LB. Liver disease in pregnancy. N Engl J Med 1996; **335:** 569-76.

Lunzer M, Barnes P, Byth K, O'Halloran M. Serum bile acid concentrations during pregnancy and their relationship to obstetric cholestasis. Gastroenterology 1986; **91:** 825-9.

Reyes H. The spectrum of liver and gastrointestinal disease seen in cholestasis of pregnancy. Gastroenterol Clin North Am 1992; **21:** 905-21.

Riely CA. Acute fatty liver of pregnancy. Semin Liver Dis 1987; **7:** 47-54.

Rustgi VK, Hoofmagle JH. Viral hepatitis during pregnancy. Semin Liver Dis 1987; **7:** 40-6.

Chapter 9

Pre- and Post-transplant assessment

INTRODUCTION

For many years, following the first attempts in the 1960s, liver transplantation was considered to be a last-ditch procedure when all other medical or surgical interventions had failed. However, with the advances in donor organ preservation, surgical techniques and control of rejection that have been made over the past 10-15 years it has become a viable treatment option for many patients with end-stage chronic liver disease or acute liver failure. One year survival rates of 80-90% are now achieved in low risk recipients. Even in acute liver failure, despite the critical state of the patients, 70-75% may be expected to survive. Indeed, there are now hundreds of patients around the world who have survived more than five years (some more than 20 years) after receiving liver grafts and the number of long-term survivors is increasing rapidly. In addition to 'standard' (whole organ) orthotopic liver transplantation, advances that have been made in surgical techniques include: i) auxillary ('piggyback') grafting for acute liver failure, where the patient's liver is left in situ and the graft takes over its functions, and is usually later removed when the recipient's own liver recovers, or can be left in situ without immunosuppresant cover; ii) 'split-liver' transplantation, in which one donor organ is divided and grafted into two (sometimes three) recipients, and occasionally, iii) living-related donor transplantation (usually parent to child), in which (normally) the smaller (left) lobe of the donor's liver is used. However, a key factor in the dramatic improvement in survival has been the increased knowledge and understanding that has been gained over the years about i) which patients are most likely to benefit from transplantation, ii) improved anaesthetic and peri-operative management and iii) the requirements for monitoring and clinical management of patients, both in the immediate post-operative period and long-term.

PRE-TRANSPLANT ASSESSMENT

Selection of patients who are likely to benefit from a liver graft requires careful clinical judgement based both on the prognosis and on the quality of life with regard to the primary illness. The criteria are complex and depend on the aetiology of the liver failure and whether it is acute or is a consequence of long-standing chronic liver disease. The overall condition of the patient to withstand such a major surgical procedure needs to be carefully assessed. Haemodynamic and respiratory status, patency of major blood vessels and concomitant diseases are essential considerations. The potential effects of the immunosuppressive drug therapy (to prevent graft rejection) on disease recurrence (e.g., in patients transplanted for malignant disorders or viral hepatitis) or on other complications such as pre-existing renal disease also need to be considered.

In contrast to other solid organ grafting, pre-transplant tissue typing of recipients for HLA matching is not an essential requirement, except when combined transplants (e.g., liver and kidney) are being performed, because the liver appears to be an 'immunologically privileged' organ and donor-recipient incompatibility leading to hyperacute rejection is a rare event (see below). It is thought that this is because hepatocytes, which comprise the mass of the liver, do not normally express HLA Class II antigens and express Class I only relatively weakly. Nonetheless, recipients are usually HLA typed so that the data are available in the event of development of post-transplant complications including, occasionally, graft-versus-host disease.

ACUTE LIVER FAILURE (ALF)
By definition, transplantation for ALF is performed as an emergency procedure and early assessment of the need for a transplant is required. The rate of onset of the illness is an important indicator of the likely outcome. Paradoxically, those with hyperacute ALF, i.e., with the most rapid development of encephalopathy (Chapter 1), have the greatest chance of a spontaneous recovery. However, aetiology also has a considerable influence on outcome. The best prognosis is seen in cases of acute fatty liver of pregnancy (Chapter 8) and the worst in sub-acute ALF due to non-A, non-B viral infections, Wilson disease and in the rare cases of acute presentations of autoimmune hepatitis. Thus, different sets of criteria apply in different patients (Figure 9.1).

Coagulation factors are perhaps the most sensitive indicators of hepatic function (Chapter 1) and are widely used in assessing the severity of liver injury. In ALF due to deliberate or accidental paracetamol (acetaminophen) overdose a rise in the prothrombin time (INR) 3-4 days after the overdose indicates a poor prognosis while a fall at that time is associated with a high rate of spontaneous recovery. The development of a metabolic acidosis and hyperlactataemia is a poor prognostic sign. Other indicators of a poor prognosis include rising plasma creatinine concentration (indicating incipient renal failure) and progression to grade III or IV encephalopathy (Chapter 1). The plasma bilirubin concentration is not a particularly useful index in this situation, or in hyperacute ALF due to other causes because, due to the rapid development of the condition, there is often insufficient time for the bilirubin to rise to very high concentrations. In acute or sub-acute ALF, however, the bilirubin concentration is an important prognostic determinant, along with age and evidence of coagulopathy (Figure 9.1).

Indications for liver transplantation in acute liver failure (ALF)	
Paracetamol-induced ALF	**Other causes of ALF**

Arterial pH < 7.3 [a]
 	
or all of the following: [a]
  prothrombin time > 100 secs
      (INR > 8)
  Creatinine > 300 μmol/L
  Grade III/IV encephalopathy
	Prothrombin time > 100 secs (INR > 8) [a]
	
	or any three of the following: [a]
	  Age < 10 or > 40 years
	  Aetiology: Non-A, non-B viral infection
	      or halothane or other drugs
	  Jaundice to encephalopathy time > 7 days
	  Prothrombin time > 50 secs (INR > 4)
	
	or: [b]
	  Age < 30 years + factor V < 20%
	  or age > 30 years + factor V < 30%

Figure 9.1 Indications for liver transplantation in patients with paracetamol-induced and other causes of acute liver failure. Adapted from a) O'Grady et al, Gastroenterology 1989; 97: 439-445 and b) Bernuau et al, Hepatology 1986; 6: 648-651 with permission

Hypoglycaemia, due to increased circulating insulin, impaired gluconeogenesis and an inability to mobilise glycogen stores, can develop rapidly and blood glucose concentrations should therefore be monitored at hourly intervals. Hypophosphataemia and hypomagnesaemia are also common findings that require correction.

CHRONIC LIVER DISEASE
In selecting patients with advanced chronic liver disease for liver transplantation there are the advantages that there is usually more time to make the assessment and to take measures to improve their general state of health prior to the operation. Projected life expectancy and quality of life if a transplant is not performed are the two major considerations. Again, as with ALF, aetiology of the primary liver disease is a determining factor and different criteria apply in different conditions. The number of chronic liver diseases for which liver transplantation is a viable treatment option is now large and a comprehensive review is beyond the scope of this book. Thus, only the major disease groups will be considered here.

CHOLESTATIC LIVER DISEASES

Biliary atresia, in which there is failure of the bile ducts to develop normally, accounts for the majority of children receiving liver transplants in most centres. The diagnosis and management of this rare congenital abnormality requires highly specialised expertise. Early recognition of the ominous significance of conjugated hyperbilirubinaemia in an infant who otherwise looks well, and urgent intervention, are essential. Usually a portoenterostomy (Kasai procedure), involving a surgical bypass of the bile ducts by joining a loop of the intestine directly to the liver, is first performed. If this fails, a transplant is the only option. Pre-transplant assessment is based mainly on clinical criteria.

In adults, the two chronic cholestatic liver diseases for which liver transplantation is most frequently performed are primary biliary cirrhosis (PBC) and primary sclerosing cholangitis (PSC) (see Chapter 6). Patients with PBC represent one of the easiest groups of patients in which to define the timing of transplantation (Figure 9.2). In these patients, the plasma bilirubin concentration has been recognised to be an excellent prognostic marker. Once concentrations exceed 170 µmol/l, the estimated life-expectancy without a transplant is 18 months. As with other forms of cholestatic liver disease, hepatocyte function is usually well preserved and the plasma albumin concentration and prothrombin time remain normal until late stage disease. Occasionally, where the patient's quality of life has deteriorated significantly, for example if they have severe intractable pruritus (itching), transplants are performed earlier. A number of prognostic models for PBC have been developed. The most commonly used are the European and Mayo Clinic models, which take account of a large number of variables including the patient's age, plasma bilirubin and albumin concentrations, prothrombin time, and various clinical and histological parameters. Although these and other models have been validated for groups of patients, the confidence limits are wide and they are not usually applied for timing transplantation for the individual patient.

The timing of liver transplantation for PSC is much more difficult because of the fluctuating course of the disease, complications relating to concomitant ulcerative colitis (which is frequently associated with PSC), and the unpredictability of the development of cholangiocarcinoma. The latter is a fairly frequent late complication of PSC and carries a poor prognosis after transplantation because of early distant tumour recurrence. Unfortunately, there are no diagnostic tumour markers for cholangiocarcinoma and asymptomatic tumours are difficult to diagnose even with cytological examination of brushings of the biliary tract obtained by cholangiography. Thus sustained or progressive jaundice and clinical judgement determine the timing of transplantation in these patients (Figure 9.2).

Liver transplantation in primary biliary cirrhosis or primary sclerosing cholangitis	
Primary biliary cirrhosis	**Primary sclerosing cholangitis**
Plasma bilirubin > 170 µmol/L Significant deterioration in quality of life (e.g., severe intractable pruritis)	Sustained progressive elevations in serum bilirubin in the absence of cholangiographic evidence of a dominant bile duct stricture or cholangiocarcinoma. Weight loss, muscle wasting and evidence of decompensation (e.g., intractable ascites) Recurrent life-threatening variceal haemorrhage not responding to sclerotherapy.

Figure 9.2 Indications for considering liver transplantation in patients with primary biliary cirrhosis or primary sclerosing cholangitis

OTHER CHRONIC LIVER DISORDERS

Patients with other chronic liver diseases who require liver transplantation for the development of acute or subacute liver failure have been considered earlier. This section deals with transplantation for advanced, end-stage cirrhosis - most frequently due to chronic viral hepatitis, alcoholic liver disease (ALD), autoimmune hepatitis (AIH), or of unknown cause (cryptogenic cirrhosis). The prime indications for transplantation in these cases are evidence of developing hepatic decompensation and encephalopathy, intractable complications (such as difficulty in controlling bleeding from oesophageal or gastric varices) associated with long-standing cirrhosis, and significantly diminishing quality of life. At this stage the liver is often shrunken and, due to the large reduction in numbers of surviving hepatocytes, plasma aminotransferases are often not markedly elevated. But progressively increasing plasma bilirubin concentrations and prothrombin times usually indicate a poor prognosis. Attempts have been made to develop prognostic models based on plasma biochemical and other parameters but these have not proved to be particularly useful for the individual patient and decisions to transplant are normally based on overall clinical judgement.

A major consideration in these cases is whether or not there is underlying malignancy. Hepatocellular carcinoma (HCC) is a common sequel of long-standing cirrhosis, particularly in cirrhosis due to chronic hepatitis B or C. The high rate of recurrence of this tumour following transplantation, possibly accelerated by the immunosuppressive therapy required, and the consequent poor post-transplant prognosis has led to a fall in the numbers of patients with HCC who are transplanted. Patients with one small (< 4 cm diameter) discrete tumour have the best chance of survival. Plasma alpha-fetoprotein (AFP) measurements are part of the standard pre-transplant assessement but are not always reliable because patients with small tumours often have AFP concentrations within the normal range and even quite large tumours can be 'AFP-negative'. Thus radiological investigations are normally undertaken to establish the size, number and precise locations of any tumours.

Additional important pre-transplant considerations apply in patients with cirrhosis due to chronic viral hepatitis or alcohol. In cases of chronic hepatitis B or C, there is a high rate of viral persistence or re-infection after grafting and careful pre-transplant assessment of the stage and status of the patient's infection needs to be made by testing for appropriate viral markers (Chapter 3). The use of antiviral therapy before and after the operation also needs to be considered and, since some of the immunosuppressive drugs (especially corticosteroids) used to prevent graft rejection enhance viral replication, the post-transplant drug regimen requires careful planning. Patients with alcoholic cirrhosis require complex pre-transplant evaluation. At the outset, an assessment of whether the patient is only an alcohol abuser or is actually alcohol dependent needs to be made. The distinction is more than academic, since alcohol abusers are more likely to be able to stop drinking and appear to have an excellent prognosis with sustained abstinence after transplantation. Extensive medical assessment is required also to determine whether there are any neurological, cardiological, nutritional, or other complications (which are common in excessive alcohol consumers) that are contraindications to, or require correction before, transplantation. A prognostic index, the Clinical and Laboratory Index (CCLI), employing routinely available laboratory information to derive a score that is predictive of the one-year mortality is used to assess the need for transplantation in patients with alcoholic cirrhosis in some centres. The CCLI incorporates 12 clinical and laboratory variables including age, prothrombin time, plasma bilirubin and albumin concentrations, plasma alkaline phosphatase activity, nutritional status and various clinical and histological findings. Alternatively, the Child-Pugh classification (Chapter 1) may be used, although this is not specific for alcoholic liver disease.

POST-TRANSPLANT ASSESSMENT

EARLY POST-OPERATIVE PERIOD

The quality of the functioning of the graft immediately after transplantation is a major determinant of the future clinical course and is consequently of great importance. Primary non-function of the graft, i.e., a liver that does not appear to work satisfactorily from the outset, is usually due to the poor quality of the donor organ. Hyperacute rejection has been described but is a very rare cause of immediate graft failure. Its differentiation from primary non-function is difficult but may be suspected if the graft appears to work initially during the first 6-24 hours only to then fail.

The standard biochemical liver tests have little value during the immediate post-operative period because the patient's blood will have been extensively diluted by multiple transfusions during the operation. Plasma aminotransferase activities on the second post-operative day are more reliable and are almost always elevated. This represents so-called 'preservation injury' to the donor organ acquired during its removal from the donor, and subsequent preservation and transportation prior to transplant. Thereafter, a progressive fall in the AST/ALT activities (ideally in decrements of 30-50% of the previous day's value) indicates good graft function, while persistently high concentrations suggest that the graft is not functioning well. Some authorities are of the opinion that plasma α-glutathione-S-transferase (GST-α) activities are a more sensitive indicator of graft function during this period (as well as in the longer term) than the standard aminotransferases but others have not found GST-α to be more useful than AST/ALT. The plasma bilirubin concentration is the least useful of these parameters, although falling concentrations are an encouraging sign of good graft function.

Other parameters that are essential for monitoring graft function post-operatively are the blood hydrogen ion concentration, glucose and coagulation factors. There is almost always hyperglycaemia during the very early post-operative phase but, with normal graft function, the blood glucose usually normalises over the following 24-48 hours and there is a decreasing requirement for insulin. Persistence of the hyperglycaemia despite increasing doses of insulin indicates poor graft function. For the reasons given above, measurement of coagulation factors in the immediate post-operative period do not give an accurate assessment of graft function but their reliability increases during the following 2-7 days. Occasionally, an isolated rise in prothrombin time (INR) may be observed but this appears to have no significant implications. However, a continuously rising INR together with rising blood hydrogen ion concentration (suggesting the development of a metabolic acidosis) and persistent hyperglycaemia is indicative of poor graft function. The quality and quantity of bile produced by the graft and the rapidity with which the patient metabolises anaesthetic and sedative drugs are additional useful parameters for monitoring graft function.

Acute cellular rejection, requiring increased immunosuppressive therapy for control, occurs in 50-70% of cases during the first three weeks after transplantation, with a peak prevalence at about the 7th day. The diagnosis of acute rejection is suggested by deterioration in the above parameters but there is no consensus on which is the most reliable. The INR is usually only minimally raised.Daily monitoring will often demonstrate an abrupt increase in plasma aminotransferase activities (but seldom > 10-fold) and plasma bilirubin concentrations, with less marked elevations of alkaline phosphatase and gamma-glutamyltransferase. An increasing plasma bilirubin concentration seems to be the most sensitive indicator but rising aminotransferases appear to be more specific. However, liver histology is required to confirm acute rejection. Serious derangement of the biochemical liver tests, particularly very marked elevations of plasma aminotransferase activity in conjunction with evidence of a coagulopathy, is highly suggestive of problems with the vascular supply to the graft.

INTERMEDIATE FOLLOW-UP

Management of patients during the months following a liver transplant involves frequent monitoring of biochemical liver tests for signs of late acute or chronic rejection, and frequent microbiological surveillance for evidence of infections. Late acute rejection, occurring more than one month after transplantation, is diagnosed similarly to early acute rejection. Chronic rejection is suspected if the biochemical liver tests have previously been generally normal but begin to become deranged. In this situation, the aminotransferases and INR may be only mildly elevated but there is a progressive increase in the plasma bilirubin and other cholestatic indicators. These changes can also be seen in fungal, bacterial and viral infections, to which the immunosuppressed patient is particularly susceptible, but can usually be differentiated from rejection episodes on clinical and histological criteria together with microbiological investigations. De novo, or more often reactivation of latent, infections with cytomegalovirus (CMV), as well as herpes simplex (HSV) and varicella zoster (VZV) viruses, are a frequent post-transplant complication. CMV is the single most important infection in transplant recipients and is potentially life-threatening. HSV reactivates during the first 1-3 weeks and about one third of patients develop clinical evidence of the infection. VZV infection in adults is usually a reactivation (primary infections are commoner in children), occurring later and less predictably than with other viruses, and typically presents as shingles affecting a single site. Special considerations apply to the management of patients transplanted for chronic hepatitis B and C. Due to the high rate of viral re-infection (see above), careful monitoring of plasma HBV-DNA or HCV-RNA is required to detect viral reactivation and provide information on which to base anti-viral treatment strategies. If anti-HBs immunoglobulin is being used to suppress HBV, titres of this antibody will also need to be monitored.

During this period also, patients are generally metabolically unstable and require careful adjustment of their immunosuppression. The principal immunosuppressive drugs used are glucocorticoids, azathioprine, cyclosporin and tacrolimus (FK506) in various combinations or, in the case of the latter two agents, increasingly frequently as monotherapy. Glucocorticoids and azathioprine are usually administered in standard doses which are adjusted on the basis of clinical criteria. However, cyclosporin and tacrolimus are nephrotoxic and potentially neurotoxic at high doses. Their metabolism is affected by a number of factors, including graft function and other drugs such as corticosteroids or antibiotics that may be required, which may variably increase or decrease the blood concentrations at given doses. Thus, frequent monitoring (at least two or three times per week) of blood concentrations of these two drugs is required during the months following transplantation in order to maintain concentrations within a fairly narrow therapeutic range that provides adequate immunosuppression with minimal toxicity.

LONG-TERM MONITORING

From the laboratory standpoint, long-term monitoring of liver transplant recipients is relatively straightforward, unless complications arise. By one year, most patients are well stabilised and require only three-monthly check-ups with routine biochemical liver tests and haematological investigations. By this time also, they are usually well established on their maintenance immunosuppressive drug regimens and much less frequent monitoring of cyclosporin or tacrolimus concentrations is required. Late graft loss, occurring more than one year after transplantation, is relatively rare and today many such cases can be rescued with a second transplant. The commonest causes of late graft failure are uncontrollable chronic rejection and recurrence of the primary disease. Recurrence of hepatitis B and C, and of malignancy in patients transplanted for hepatic tumours, has been discussed above. However, as in other solid organ transplantation there is an increased risk of non-hepatic malignancies, particularly lymphomas, arising either de novo or through reactivation by immunosuppression of extrahepatic tumours that have previously been apparently successfully treated. As the numbers of long-term survivors rises, recurrence of PBC and AIH following transplantation is being seen with increasing frequency. With AIH, this may be due partly to current practice to reduce immunosuppressive therapy to very low concentrations, or gradually wean patients off the drugs altogether, in the longer term.

FURTHER READING

The Practice of Liver Transplantation. Williams R, Portmann B, Tan K-C, eds. Churchill Livingstone, Edinburgh; 1995.

INDEX